TRADITIONAL WESTERN
HERBAL MEDICINE

TRADITIONAL WESTERN HERBAL MEDICINE
As Above So Below

Elisabeth Brooke

AEON

First published in 2019 by
Aeon Books Ltd
12 New College Parade
Finchley Road
London NW3 5EP

British Library Cataloguing in Publication Data

A C.I.P. for this book is available from the British Library

ISBN-13: 978-1-91159-720-9

Typeset by Medlar Publishing Solutions Pvt Ltd, India
Printed and bound in Great Britain by TJ International Ltd

www.aeonbooks.co.uk

For
Magical Herbalists
everywhere

As above
So below
As within
So without
As the Universe
So the Soul

The laws of physic are agreeable to the laws of nature. Physic imitates nature. Its design is, to preserve the body in health, to defend it from infirmity, to strengthen and invigorate the weak, and to raise the dejected. (Culpeper, 1798, p. xiii)

The vegetable world, with its occult virtues and power, is, of all others, the sublimist subject for the exertion of genius and afford the highest gratification to a benevolent mind: since there are no infirmities incident to our fallen nature that it does not enable us to alleviate or remove. (Culpeper, 1798, p. xiv)

CONTENTS

PART TWO: THE PRACTICE

ACKNOWLEDGEMENTS

Firstly, thanks to Melinda McDougall and Oliver Rathbone for asking me to write this book and publishing my backlist. To the women of the Magical Herbalism and Astrology and Medicine workshops. Particular thanks to Joanna Watters and the participants of the Astrology and Herbs intensive in Lefkas, Greece, who worked through my ideas on Temperaments and Herbs and gave me many valuable insights and very helpful feedback. To Maggie Hyde and Geoffrey Cornelius of the Company of Astrologers, where I learned and later taught Traditional Astrology and Decumbiture. To the librarians of The Classical Association Library, The Welcome Library for the History of Medicine and the British Library for their help in sourcing the material and to the libraries themselves for being there; what an extraordinary resource they are, and how lucky we are to have them. To Duncan Barford for his meticulous editing and Cecily Blench of Aeon Books for her help.

INTRODUCTION

This book traces the parallel history of astrology and medicine from Ancient Greece, through the Renaissance to the twentieth and twenty-first centuries. Astrology was a companion to medicine for the ancients. It was obvious that the seasons affected health, overheating in summer, phlegm and chills in winter. The phases of the moon would also be seen to affect people, emotions were heightened at the full moon, and wounds were inclined to bleed more, while fevers peaked.

On the island of Cos, in the fourth century BCE, the medical school of Hippocrates was close to the astrological school of Berosus and we can imagine there was contact and discourse between the schools. In the first century CE, Galen the physician and Ptolemy the astrologer were contemporaries of equal renown. Eclipsed in Europe after the fall of the Roman Empire, both writers' works were preserved and commented on by Arab and Byzantine scholars, until they were returned to Europe in the fourteenth century after the fall of the Byzantine Empire. Taken up by the new universities, medicine and astrology once more became inseparable.

This culminated in the high point of astrological medicine, in the seventeenth century with the work of William Lilly and Nicholas Culpeper, another pair of friends. Both men practiced the astrology of

divination, *katarche* and herbal medicine. They used their arts to promote the Parliamentary cause during the Civil War. Lilly was better
connected than Culpeper, who was more radical. Culpeper champi-
oned the cause of popular medicine and unleashed a Pandora's box of
hostility from the College of Physicians.

After the enlightenment discoveries of Hooke, Harvey et al. astrological medicine slipped from view never to recover its former place
at the heart of healing and instead became an object of derision and
ridicule. Medicine remained herbal until the development of modern
chemistry in the twentieth century, at least in the cities of Europe; in the
countryside herbal medicine continued until the development of the
National Health Service.

Dissatisfaction with chemical medicine has meant renewed interest herbal medicine. Astrology also is more mainstream these days;
however, the re-uniting of the two has been resisted strongly. This is
especially odd as both Traditional Chinese Medicine and Ayurvedic
medicine have their parallel astrological systems, which are accepted
or tolerated. The English tradition is not viewed so leniently. "Oriental
systems" might have philosophies as exotic as they wished, because
they were "other" and not expected to be rational. This, I believe, is an
expression of what Edward Said (1978) called "orientalism", the practice of both patronising and culturally appropriating "exotic" belief
systems, which are "indigestible" in some way in Western culture. By
exoticizing medical astrology, it becomes "other" and therefore neutral-
ized and acceptable within Western culture.

There is a lack of confidence in Western herbalism, let alone herbalism and astrology, that dark corner of divination. Many herbalists wishing for a philosophical framework to pin their practice on, choose one of
these "oriental" disciplines to give them structure and authority, while
the English tradition of Culpeper and Lilly remains hidden and forgotten. Why is the practice of astrology so unacceptable, when *shen* or *gui*
or *qi* or *prana* are not controversial?[1]

I suspect the reason is a cultural memory we have in Britain of the
consequences of practising the magical and esoteric, the witch panics of
the sixteenth and seventeenth centuries. The common view of witches
was that they were crazy old hags, illiterate and credulous. The reality was different; many were healers, midwives, astrologers, hedge

---

[1]*Shen, gui* and *qi* are from Traditional Chinese Medicine, and *prana* is from Ayurveda.

witches, and cunning folk, denounced by the emboldened College of Physicians and Protestant church who wished to regularise and control lay people, especially women, and prevent them from encroaching into their sphere of influence (Brooke, 1993, pp. 83–92).

Although, England and Scotland did not kill "witches" on a scale comparable to other European countries, the *fear* of witchcraft became embedded in our psyche as the ultimate sanction for radicality. Culpeper was charged with this crime because he was both translating medical texts into English, which undermined the power and incomes of the College of Physicians, and ridiculing their medical skill and greed (speaking truth to power).

As British herbalists we enjoy a freedom to practice unknown in most Western countries. I believe in response we have signed a Faustian pact to be "scientific" and reject half of our European Tradition so as to "not rock the boat" by using anything which smacks of witchery and revolution. Most British herbalists, including myself, trained in a tradition founded in Physiomedicalism, introduced from the USA in the nineteenth century. Physiomedicalism was a Protestant tradition which incorporated settler medicine and Native American herbalism, with the Protestant doctrines predominating. This system has latterly fallen out of favour and science-based medicine has replaced it. This leaves the British practice adrift, without a philosophical framework. However, for many this is a preferable situation than embracing the English tradition and being seen as a "wizard".[2]

Those of us who have put our heads above the parapet[3] have been barely tolerated and generally marginalized. It is twenty-six years since I published *A Woman's Book of Herbs* (Brooke, 2018), and a lot has changed in the world of herbal medicine. "Energetics" (a term borrowed from Traditional Chinese Medicine) has become acceptable. It is a term that sanitizes the magical nature of herbs, and provides a language which does not offend or confront. Even so, that the message of the deep, wide, wisdom of nature is spreading wider and gaining traction among biologists as well as herbalists can only be good news for ourselves as users of herbal medicine and for the planet, for never has it been more

---

[2]My personal experience in general practice was that about fifty per cent of patients, were relieved I did not have a cauldron bubbling in the corner and a broomstick by the door, and fifty per cent were disappointed I did not.

[3]Graeme Tobyn, Dylan Warren-Davis.

urgent that we recognize, value, cherish, and protect our natural world. (See Macfarlane, 2016.)

The dark forces of greed, big pharma and ignorance remain powerful and, through a corrupt media, continue to attack natural medicine on spurious grounds.[4] It was the same in Culpeper's day. His translation of the *London Pharmacopoeia* into a language accessible to non-professionals was met by furious opposition, including a false charge of witchcraft against him. The penalty for witchcraft was a grisly death, by fire or drowning, so the College of Physicians, perhaps like today's big Pharma, anxious to maintain their monopoly over medical treatment and indifferent to the fate of those whose could not afford their fees, was prepared to kill rather than share their knowledge. History was on Culpeper's side; his book, the *New English Physician* has never been out of print.

Despite opposition, ridicule and threats, herbal medicine enjoys continued and growing support. In recent years there have been programmes to bring herbal medicine to people who are marginalised (refugees, the homeless, and those on low incomes) and to question the power imbalance inherent in the practitioner-patient relationship, exploring new ways to offer healing. These include: Radical Herbalism, Herbalists Without Borders, and Grass Roots Remedies.

In the section on planets and herbs I cover herbs not discussed in *A Woman's Book of Herbs* (Brooke, 2018). There are many old favourites, beloved herbs that I have worked with for over forty years, others are new friends that I am getting to know. The breadth and depth of plant life means no one can fully learn all the plants available. We all self-select those remedies which appeal to us, those we can pick and prepare easily, or those introduced to us by colleagues and friends.

In "Decumbiture" (below, p. 125) I discuss the singularity of the decumbiture chart, as an individual symbolic representation of the therapeutic relationship between client and practitioner, understanding its symbolism as radical for this moment of meeting (or falling sick).

---

[4]As I write, the *Guardian* newspaper runs a scare story about possible interactions of herbs and pharmaceuticals (Devlin, 2018), and a lecture (Wellcome Collection, 2018), on Ayurvedic remedies by pharmacists, warns of the dangers of "untested" remedies while simultaneously noting the mild side effects found in a study (headache, stomach ache, diarrhoea, etc.) whereas pharmaceuticals for similar conditions caused serious side effects including diabetes! Both examples show the prejudice of science and the group-think we have been fed that science=good, alternative=bad. For this book I tried without success to find the figures for iatrogenic deaths caused by doctors and mainstream medicine, but these were not available.

In a similar way, I believe the plants we chose, the way we use them, and the clients that come to us, are individual and specific to the practitioner, the patient, and the plant. By this I mean that I, as an individual, will be attracted to certain herbs, or to different herbs at different times. I may be thinking a lot about a particular herb and this may attract to me several patients who will benefit from taking that plant.

This happens so often as to be commonplace. The energy I am putting out, by thinking about the plant, draws to me a particular patient who is attracted to my energy, which resonates with something within them that needs what I offer. It is possible that one stage further back the plant calls to me. I notice it for the first time when people in my circle talk about the plant, or events in the news make me think of the plant, or I see pictures of the plant, and this calling is answering a need I have in me to get to know the plant and learn the lesson it has to teach me and to use it with my patients.

Basic information about the plants can be learned, but we need to use our other senses to choose which liver remedy to use, which skin remedy, why Dandelion and not Milk Thistle, Valerian or Lettuce. This requires a subtler understanding of the plant. Long-experienced herbalists I know, will say, "use this remedy, not that one" for a certain condition, but will often not have the language to explain why it should be so. Of course, there is the light of experience, but I contend there is also a deep knowing of the nature of the plant, which may go beyond language to the world of symbols, feelings and intuitions. I discussed this at length in *A Woman's Book of Herbs* all those years ago.

Because recently in the UK many herbal trainings are conducted in university science departments, the knowledge of the subtle energies in practice risks being lost. There is a danger that by attempting to be "acceptable" to medical science, we lose those very subtleties that make herbal remedies superior to active principles extracted in a lab. The scientific paradigm also has the double negative of removing the practitioner from the equation and reducing plant actions to a tick-box list of active principles.

The mystery of the practitioner-client relationship, the multi-faceted properties of plants and the wonder of healing are lost. Of course, in time, a sensitive practitioner will appreciate the singularity of the practitioner-patient interaction and recognise the subtleties of plant medicine and be drawn to or turned off by particular plants. However, this may take many years. If each neophyte herbalist were to sit with a plant and get to know it, *really* get to know it, they would transform their understanding of the nature of the plant and of themselves, their learning and healing path.

For the plants give generously. They will reveal layer upon layer of their mysteries and wisdom, which lead us beyond the limits we have placed on our creativity and sensitivity. I began working this way with plants by complete accident. I had trained in the scientific way and indeed had taught pharmacology and pathology and differential diagnosis to herbal students for several years. I had also studied astrology and had done some psychic development work. I ran a small group, mainly comprised of alternative practitioners, which would meet up monthly to talk about plants. One morning I had the idea to see what would happen if we tuned into the plants psychically.

The results were fantastic, and we began meeting regularly, and then another group was formed, and another. Eventually the material was collated into a book and published. My herbal colleagues were appalled and embarrassed and I was basically ostracised by the herbal community for dragging what they were trying to make scientific and acceptable into witchcraft and weirdness.

As I said at the beginning, things have changed over the last twenty-six years and thankfully some parts of the community have embraced a more holistic and sensitive way to practice herbal medicine.

My original book was so large it had to be divided into sections. The first part became *A Woman's Book of Herbs* (Brooke, 2018), the second *Women Healers Through History* (Brooke, 1993). For the third part I could not find a publisher, and it languished in a dusty corner until I was invited to write a book for Aeon Books. I decided to revive and rewrite the final part of my original book, and this is it, the third part of my original vision to show how, as healers, we have a context (our history); deep, spiritual wisdom (our herbs); and a workable philosophy (humoral medicine), which encapsulates the maxim, "as above, so below":

> there is indisputably an innate and occult virtue infused in all sublunary things, animal, vegetable and mineral by the actions of the heavenly bodies upon the ambient and elementary matter which produces the astonishing variety in Nature which is infinitely beyond our knowledge and comprehension. (Sibly, in Culpeper, 1798, pp. viii–ix)

PART ONE

THEORY

Fire

Fire meditation

Imagine you are sitting in front of a candle flame, you feel safe and warm. Allow your gaze to rest on the flame. Watch it as it bends and sways with the breeze. Feel the warmth on your face. Watch the light shimmer around it. Then slowly, gently, allow yourself to merge with the flame. It will not burn you but gently envelop you with warmth and light. Be aware of your physical body. How does it feel to be surrounded by fire? Take a moment to sense the flames as they enclose you and notice any changes in your heart or your skin or other organs of the body. Then allow the fire to pass through your whole body. Feel yourself enveloped by warm, healing fire. How does this make you feel emotionally? Register and remember any feelings it brings up and then let them go. Be aware of any images or memories which come up. Notice them and let them go. Then notice how fire affects your mind and your thoughts. How does your mind react in the presence of fire? Take a moment to let the thoughts run by you without judgement or questions. Slowly separate yourself from the flame and return to watching the candle. Gently come back into the room.[1]

---

[1]You may wish to pre-record this and the other meditations and play them while you do the meditation.

The most favoured current theory of how our world began centres around the Big Bang theory. The Big Bang Theory states, using mathematical models, that 13.8 billion years ago a "small singularity" expanded. A second after this expansion the surrounding heat was 5.5 billion Celsius. After this expansion the universe cooled sufficiently to form sub-atomic particles and later atoms. Giant clouds of these primordial elements coalesced through gravity in haloes of dark matter and eventually formed the stars and galaxies. Most of the atoms formed by the Big Bang were hydrogen and helium and some lithium. Whereas simple atomic nuclei formed within three minutes of the big bang, thousands of years passed before the first electrically neutral atoms were formed.

The Big Bang was not an explosion in space, but an explosion of space. The Big Bang Theory does not describe the origin of the universe, because energy, time and space existed before the Big Bang. Neither does the Big Bang Theory account for the cause of the density and high temperature of the initial state of the universe. It does explain how life as we understand it began; after the initial episode, the heavier elements were synthesised within stars or supernovae. We then, are stardust.

To recap: before the Big Bang there was order of a kind, as energy, time and space already existed. For some reason there was a "conflict moment" (O' Donohue, 2010, p. 93) and then an explosion. This image of massive heat and transformation encapsulates the essence of fire. Empedocles writing in the fifth century BCE postulated that a spinning mass of fire flew off from the sun, cooled, and formed the earth. The steamy atmosphere of the earth then cooled and separated into gases or air and the shallow oceans (Gullan-Whur, 1987, p. 20). As the universe cooled, atoms and the elements were formed, and after time physical matter developed.

Keywords for fire: it initiates, explodes and heats. It has the qualities of action, energy, and power. Fire leads, explores, is fearless, assertive, and dynamic. Heat scorches, burns, melts, radiates, invigorates, shines, spotlights and sends out sparks, brings life to matter.

Physical fire: is expressed as burns, fevers, inflammation, drying, overheating, restlessness, burn-out, irritation, angry wounds, boils, rashes, and eruptions.

Fire psychology: is self-willed, self-actualising, selfish, hasty, aggressive and passionate. Fire is intuitive; it picks up ideas and acts on them. Fire is visionary, it is the genius which interrupts and disrupts. Fire does not obey reason (Air), consider practical results (Earth), or respond to feelings (Water), but follows hunches pursuing its desire (Gullan-Whur, 1987, p. 23).

Fire emotionally: represents experience centred in personal identity (Arroyo, 1978, p. 95). Fire gives a strong self-belief, a measure of impersonality, enthusiasm, energy, self-centredness and a desire for freedom. Fire is joyful and warm-hearted. Fire can direct its will consciously.

Negative fire: shows as egomania, cruelty, bullying, selfishness, rashness, intolerance, impatience, restlessness.

Weak fire: is expressed as low energy and a tendency towards depression and despondency. Weak fire is experienced as a lack of joy and distrust of life because of pessimism, and a lack of self-confidence. Weak fire has difficulty in beginning anything, lacks the creative spark to initiate and find the energy for action. It is expressed as conservatism, meanness, sadness, negativity, and fearfulness.

Spiritually: Fire is also spirit, the cosmic fire, the divine spark. Fire is said to rule the etheric or vital body which transforms the elements of Air and Water to support the functions of the physical body. In Greek philosophy, Fire and Air actively and consciously form life by rising and expanding and are Apollonian, or the rational, ordered, and disciplined aspects of human nature (Arroyo, 1978, p. 93).

Social fire: O'Donohue talks about the hearth, where traditionally people gathered, where spirit was focused, refined and preserved (O'Donohue, 2010, p. 111). Today we might think of the campfire or the kitchen table, where people meet and exchange their news and where experiences are shared. Traditionally, the hearth was where tales of the past were told, the teachings of the clans were passed on, or "the fecundity of the past in conversation with the possibility of the future" (O'Donohue, 2010, p. 113). Paracelsus gave salamanders to the fire element; those magical beings that sometimes we glimpse in the heart of the flames. According to Paracelsus, salamanders are controlled by cultivating contentment and placidity, in other words, the opposite from Fire, Earth. Today the ersatz fire of the flat screen provides a sterile focal point where the tales of others, cynically constructed, imprint upon us a bogus, empty, monoculture.

A real fire excites and warms the heart as matter is transformed into smoke and ash, but Fire is also deadly. Fear of fire was used to control; the exquisite pain of a small burn, extrapolated out into the perpetual burning of hellfire, the burning alive of witches and heretics, used as a means of control and torture (O'Donohue, 2010, p. 120).

Choleric temperament

From the element comes the humour, and from the humour the temperament. Ancient authors recognised that in the same way there are four elements, there are four basic personality types. Choleric is the type for fire.

Physical characteristics

Choler, ruled by fire, is hot and dry; it makes the body lean and muscled. These are the classic athletes who have a well-developed physical body, high energy, low patience, who dislike sitting down, they will pace a room like a caged animal, finding silence and stillness almost unbearable. They will often be hot to the touch; sometimes their skin feels almost like it is burning. Heat and dryness evaporate fluid, so the pure choleric type will be lean, with no soft edges, but not bony (that is the domain of the melancholic); instead they will be sinewy, mobile, speedy. Think dancers, athletes, soldiers, cyclists, swimmers, manual workers, outdoor workers. Their lack of patience makes them more likely to be self-employed, so they can move at their own pace, and not answer to other people.

Emotional characteristics

Impatience is a key factor, sometimes expressed as frustration, sometimes as anger. Fire slices through; a pure choleric type will be brutal, cutting, dismissive of mere emotional sensitivities, they will simply not understand them, because they do not care to ruminate on their own feelings. They are people of action. They need excitement, noise, colour, change. Change, especially, is important for fire types; boredom, routine, predictability, are depressing. Fire grasps ideas and concepts from nowhere and dashes to put their vision out into the world. They are visionary, often before their time, people who scatter seeds as they pass through. Fire is not interested in nurture; that is a job for Earth. Fire's impatience impels them to ever move forwards to the new, the exciting, the innovative. If they are frustrated, choler becomes angry, and life frustrates them most of the time. Often spoiling for a fight, cholerics raise their voices or their fists, slam doors, and walk out without a backward glance. Conversely, Fire is warm and friendly; it has, at heart, good intention. Other, colder types can bask in their heat and humour and vision and optimism and hitch a ride on their energy. For Fire is nothing if not generous. Come one, come all, the choleric says, but don't hold me back, don't weigh me down, don't drown out my spark. You are with me, great, but don't tell me your fears, don't point out drawbacks, or possible hitches, because I will shake you off like a flea. I am motion, I am energy, I am life force, I am freedom. Selfish, opinionated, brusque and competitive, Fire has high expectations of themselves and others and hates slackers and apathy. The choleric is self-starting and loves a challenge, happy to share as long as they are in charge. Egoistic choleric will not tolerate competition, nor their authority being questioned; they can be ruthless and violent if crossed. They lack subtlety and can be infuriatingly dogmatic and bullying. Simplistic in their analysis they do not see or care about nuances and so can blunder into situations, pouring petrol on a fire.

In health

The choleric is strong and resilient. They enjoy high energy and are adaptable, open, and exuberant. Cholerics have a strong physical body and high stamina. They can withstand extremes of hunger and tiredness. Because their minds are untroubled by subtleties they can also withstand great mental and emotional pressure by focusing on their goal. However, because energy is finite, cholerics can over-extend themselves and burn out. Their Fire is doused by Water (emotions), smothered by Earth (matter), and blown out by Air (thoughts).

In sickness

Heat naturally causes fevers, burns up fluids, dries out tissue, inflames, irritates and excites. It causes acute, burning pains. Sharp, stabbing, cutting, radiating, chafing, stinging, rubbing, inflaming, itching are all descriptions of the symptoms of Fire and heat. Fire sicknesses are characterised by sudden onset, restlessness, anger, and irritation. Classic choleric illness includes: sudden heart attack, stroke, stomach ulcers, migraine. They are more prone to accidents due to their aggression and speed of movement.

Regimen for choleric

Cooling down and calming down are watch-words for choleric types, not that they will listen. Being headstrong is a character trait of theirs;

they feel they are invulnerable and immortal, so sickness falls heavily when it eventually arrives. Easily extinguished, Fire for all its strength and energy is vulnerable. They hate weakness, dependency, receiving help, and will push on far further than other temperaments who are in touch with their own vulnerabilities and limitations. The classic choleric drops dead of a heart attack because they will not slow down or moderate their punishing pace. They do not grow old easily; loss of autonomy is terrifying to them. They often overdo physical exercise, so punishing fitness regimes should be enquired about, as well as sometimes an unhealthy appetite for fast food and red meat and fire-water (alcoholic spirits). They will always need a challenge, so encourage them to aim for goals and milestones in their treatment plan. Suggest mentoring others, so that they feel potent and useful. Sunshine is healing to cholerics; it recharges their batteries and allows their tense bodies to relax a little. Suggest they develop the habit of drinking a lot of water to flush out the system and cool them down.

Culpeper on the choleric temperament

> [...] they are naturally quick witted, bold, no way shame-fac'd, furious, hasty, quarrelsom, fraudulent, eloqent, corragious, stout-hearted Creatures, not given to sleep much, but much given to jesting, mocking, and lying. (Culpeper, 1652, p. 54.)

Diet and exercise fitting

> A Chollerick man is oftner hurt by much fasting and much drinking than by much eating, for much fasting weakens Nature in such people, and fills the Body full of Chollerick Humors, and breedeth adust Humors, let such eat meats hard of Digestion, as Beef, Pork, & c. and leave Danties for weaker Stomachs. Moderate drinking of small Beer doth him good, for it cools the fiery heat of his Nature, moistneth the Body which is dryed by the heat of his Complexion, and relieves radical moisture, but let a man of such a Complexion fly from Wine and strong Beer as fast as he would fly from a Dragon, for they inflame the Liver, and breed burning and hectick Feavers, Choller and hot Dropsies, and bring a man to his Grave in the prime of his Age.

Much Exercise is likewise bad for Chollerick People and breeds Inslamation and adustion of Blood, the yellow Jaundice, Consumptions, Feavers, Costiveness and Agues. (Culpeper, 1652, p. 54.)

Culpeper on signs of choler abounding[2]

It shows leanness of body, costiveness [constipation], hollow eyes, anger without cause, testy disposition, yellowness of skin, bitterness of the throat, pricking pain in the head, pulse swifter and stronger than ordinary, urine high coloured and thinner and brighter, troublesome sleeps, dreams of fire, anger, lightning and fighting. (Culpeper, 1653, p. 88.)

The Fire signs ♈ ♌ ♐

Any of the planets above have their essential nature coloured by the sign they are in. There are three Fire signs: Aries, ruled by Mars, Leo ruled by the Sun, and Sagittarius ruled by Jupiter. Aries is cardinal and is action-orientated; Leo is fixed and is concerned with maintenance; and Sagittarius is mutable and is adaptable. A Mars in Aries is different from a Mars in Leo or a Mars in Sagittarius. Mars in Aries will be really dynamic (Mars plus cardinal); Mars in Leo will be more glorious (think a brilliant energy on display, fixed, not moving so much); while a Mars in Sagittarius will be hyper-sociable, a traveller through time, space and people (Mars plus mutable-expansive).

Aries ♈

Nature

Aries is the first sign of the zodiac and has the child-like energy of beginnings. The season of Aries is Spring when new shoots are bursting forth and there is an unsophisticated, raw energy and enthusiasm. Aries as the first sign often goes alone, gets there before anyone else, and then speeds off before anyone can catch up. Prone to boredom ("why can't they catch up?"), impatience ("why is everyone so slow?"), and aggression ("I'll do it my way"). They are naive and do not bother

---

[2]A temporarily acquired condition—an illness, or a temporary excess in a choleric temperament.

to think things through but are focused on action. They have tremendous energy and infectious enthusiasm.

Famous Aries

Vincent Van Gough, Casanova, Joan Crawford.

Rulerships

Aries is cardinal Fire, a masculine sign, and rules the Spring and youth.

Dignity and debility

Mars rules Aries, the Sun is exalted in Aries, Saturn is in fall in Aries (weak) and, Venus is in detriment (weak). (See Appendix 2 for a table of dignities and debilities.)

Physical

Aries shows a muscular, smallish body that is hot and dry. Aries rules the head; migraine is a Mars condition related to stress or tension causing a crippling pain which stops the person in their tracks. Aries also shows accidents, head wounds from rash actions and fighting.

Emotional

Aries will show as impatience, irritation and anger, either expressed, or not expressed and experienced as depression. There is an arrogance with Aries which often masks insecurity and a need to be liked. They are often solitaries and may be lonely. They have an endearing naivety, which if abused can turn to bitterness or depression. They are enthusiastic, but if their ebullience is crushed they can become cynical and aggressive. Aries are loyal and generous and want to believe the best about people, and for this reason they can be easily conned.

Mental

Aries is not prone to thinking ahead, but they are quick on their feet and full of ideas, expressing the intuitive function. They are prone to depression as they are optimists and life can be disappointing. Fire, especially with regard to Aries, has energy, but not resilience; if knocked down then getting back up becomes harder with age, and so they may retreat into their own little world. Routine and boredom can cause them to lash out or make reckless decisions.

Illnesses

Headache, concussion, migraine, wounds, accidents to head or face, hot fevers, burns, acne and boils. Exhaustion and burnout, both physically and mentally.

Culpeper writes: "Under Aries are all pushes, whelkes and pimples, freckles and Sun-burning in the face; polipus or noli me tangere; all diseases in the head, as head-ach of all sorts; vertigo, frenzie, litthargie, forgetfulnesse, catalepsie, apoplexie, dead palsie, coma, falling sicknesse, convulsions, cramps, madnesse, melancholy, trembling" (Culpeper, 1651a, p. 89).

Leo ♌

Nature

Leo is ruled by the Sun and loves to shine; power and adoration are their driving force. As fixed fire, Leo is less rash and intemperate than Aries, and is more concerned with status and power than freedom and self-determination.

Famous Leos

Mick Jagger, Jenifer Lopez, Bill Clinton, Barack Obama.

Dignity and debility

The Sun rules Leo, Saturn is in detriment in Leo, Leo is a fixed fire sign. It is masculine, a barren sign,[3] choleric, and hot and dry. The Sun rules summer, the choleric season.

---

[3]Lilly gives the barren signs as Gemini, Leo and Virgo, of which he says: "if the Ascendant or fifth house be of those signs … it generally represents few or no children" (Lilly, 1647, p. 89).

Physical

Leo rules the heart and circulation and the spine. Generally, they have an arresting, commanding presence and are hard to ignore, people who are warm and sociable and draw others into their orbit. They often have large eyes and round faces, with golden highlights or blonde hair. They can run to fat but have strong, solid bodies. They are usually attractive and have a light, warm quality about them.

Emotional

Leo's need to be at the centre of attention and adored can make them charming, but also demanding. Leo is a creative sign but can be destructive and hostile if they feel ignored. They are arrogant, successful, dominating, controlling, and they do not share space as much as dominate it. They are born leaders and so take failure and old age hard. They can be vindictive and cruel. They can suffer from delusions of grandeur.

Mental

While as long they get the recognition they feel they deserve, Leos will be happy. Ignored or belittled they become vengeful and bitter, argumentative and litigious. Depression and mania are other responses to perceived failures. Hurt pride, like a wounded lion, makes them dangerous; their rages are legendary and only annihilation of their enemies will satisfy their need for revenge. Their need to be the best can make them snobbish and competitive in a superficial way.

Illnesses

Leos have a strong constitution, as the heart rules the vital spirit. All diseases of the spine are under Leo as well as heart disease, palpitations, high fevers, eye disease, and some infectious diseases.
    Culpeper writes:

> [... U]nder Leo, are all diseases the heart or back is subject to, as
> qualmes and passions, palpitation, and trembling of the heart, vio-
> lent burning feavers, sore eyes, the yellow jaundies, and all diseases
> of choler, and such diseases as come of adustion of blood as the

pestilence; and I am afraid London will find this too true so soon as Saturne comes into Leo. I pray God mitigate this evill influence toward them at that time. (Culpeper, 1651a, p. 91.)

Culpeper denies what he sees as both Lilly's and Aristotle's contention that Leo rules convulsions:

[… I]t is one of old Aristotles opinions, which crept into his noddle, as he was marring Plato's Philosophy; The nerves have their originall from the braine; Convulsion is a plucking or twitching of the nerves; ergo it is a disease of the braine and not of the heart. (Culpeper, 1651a, p. 91.)

Sagittarius ♐

Nature

Sagittarius is mutable fire. It has the energy of fire but rather than be concerned with assertion (Aries), or power (Leo), Sagittarius demands freedom.

Famous Sagittarians

William Blake, Edith Piaf, Mary Queen of Scots, Beethoven, Walt Disney.

Dignity and debility

Sagittarius is ruled by Jupiter and the Sun is dignified in the sign. Mercury is in detriment in the sign. It is fiery, masculine and choleric.

Physical

Sagittarius rules the hips, thighs, and buttocks and the blood. Sagittarius are often larger than life: they can be tall, big-boned, overweight, or just powerfully built. If Aries is the sprinter, Sagittarius is the rugby player, as Jupiter gives great physical strength and stamina. They quite often have large, fleshy hips and thighs. Lilly writes: "a wel-favoured Countenance, somewhat long visage, but full and ruddy … the Stature somewhat above the middle size … a strong able body" (Lilly, 1647, p. 98).

Emotional

Sagittarius is the most optimistic of signs: friendly, outgoing, positive, energetic, collegiate, persuasive, warm-hearted, open and welcoming. They are resilient and philosophical. Sagittarius does not worry or pick over things; it moves on if things don't work out, it has tolerance of others and feels no need to change or criticise people. Its expansive nature embraces life and welcomes the new; the more the merrier is a good Sagittarian philosophy. They will fight for their beliefs, though, especially against hypocrisy and moribund convention, but in a non-aggressive way. Sagittarius will plough their own furrow despite criticism and ridicule, like William Blake or Edith Piaf.

Mental

Sagittarius is the sign of spirituality, philosophy, astrology and higher education. Sagittarius is interested in ideas which open up their world. They love physical travel, but also mental exploration. They are generally very contented people, as they don't seek to change or compete with other people, but, like all Fire signs, too much adversity can crush their indomitable spirit.

Illnesses

Sagittarius rules corruption of the blood, infections, sepsis, injuries to thighs and hips, high fevers, hot diseases. Culpeper writes that under Sagittarius are all diseases:

> [… A]s the Sciatica &c. fistulaes in those places, heat of blood, pestilentiall feavers; and take this for a generall rule, that Leo and Sagittarius signifies fall from horses, and hurts by four-footed beasts; they being both of them signes of horseman-ship; besides Sagittarius prejudiceth the body by choler, heat, fire, and intemperance in sports. (Culpeper, 1651a, p. 93.)

Earth

Earth meditation

Close your eyes. Imagine you are in a meadow. It is a warm summer's day. Your feet are bare. You feel the warm, moist earth beneath them. Take a second to feel the energy at the soles of your feet. Be aware of the top of your head, and now the soles of your feet. Be aware of how your body is perfectly balanced on the soft, yielding earth, how your weight sinks into the ground, and how the ground holds up the weight of your body in perfect balance and equilibrium. Now you sit on the earth and are aware of the strength and pliability of the earth, how it is held together by the grass and flowers, and how it holds the moisture which feeds the plants. It is teeming with life, home to plants, microbes, insects, fungi. Lie back on the earth, and feel your spine sink down into the soil. Feel your weight supported by the wide earth, which stretches as far as you can see. As you lie, feel the pulsing life of Mother earth as she enfolds and nourishes the great, green planet. Although it appears to be still, you can feel the pulse of the earth, contracting, relaxing, systole and diastole. The earth hums with slow steady energy, seemingly inert but strong and sinking, cold and dry. Slowly sink into the earth, feel the effect of the earth on your body, on your emotions, on your mind. Record any impressions or images or thoughts or feelings.

Earth is cold and dry; it has the quality of stillness. If Fire is energy, then Earth is matter or form expressed by solidity, slowness, sinking action, coolness, and drying properties. Earth holds our bodies together and gives boundaries and structure. It protects the more vulnerable organs with its hardness and stability, such as the cranium enclosing the brain, or the rib cage, the heart and liver. Earth holds the plant kingdom together; seeds germinate in the cold earth before they blossom, and the roots secure the plant and transport nourishment to the leaves and flowers and store the nutrients during the barren times. The Vernal Dam hypothesis suggests that spring ephemeral species, such as the Dog Tooth Violet, can decrease the potential loss of nutrients, especially nitrogen, due to their rapid uptake of these nutrients before the leaves of deciduous trees develop, at a time when nutrient uptake by the trees is minimal. Rapid decomposition of spring ephemeral foliage then makes these nutrients available to trees later in the spring, when they are more capable of taking up soil nutrients (Gilliam, 2007). Seemingly inert, there is activity, intelligence, communication, and order below the still and silent exterior of earth. This has been called "the wood wide web" (Macfarlane, 2016).

From nothing the earth was created. O'Donohue suggests the ferocity and desire to own land is a subconscious act of vengeance by the exiled human who knows one day his bones will be buried and absorbed into its body (O'Donohue, 2010, p. 144). The landscape gives us silence, depth, history, and a spiritual profundity which connects us to our primal, original, fertile origins. Earth is summer meadows, thick ancient forests, healing plants, the endless variety and complexity of Gaia, the earth goddess. Earth loves walking in forests or along a mountain path. Earth peels off the layers of chatter, the nonsense of manufactured materiality, and connects us with the true and beautiful material world; implacable, awe-inspiring, humbling nature. Earth holds memory: the standing stones of pre-history link us back to our cousins who lived fearfully on the land, scratching and scavenging for subsistence; our ancestors who called on the sky gods and rain gods and the soft breezes to pollinate a resistant soil.

Earth is the body of Gaia, yet we are ambivalent toward her, we small humans dwarfed by the redwoods, awestruck by the high mountains, terrified by mudslides and earthquakes. Currently, there is a battle to stop the incessant degradation of the earth, which stands mute as we plunder and abuse the plants and animals that live on it. Tree Sisters is a network that was founded to support and encourage women worldwide to organise and plant trees and restore the great forests of the tropics. Their aim is to plant one million trees per month and raise consciousness to "normalize a state of nature connectedness out of which new solutions and actions arise: we call this Feminine Nature Based Leadership" (Tree Sisters, 2010). This is a classic Earth enterprise: small, unflashy, hardworking, grassroots organising, working slowly towards a concrete goal, using existing structures and local networks, through word of mouth, to build something which is self-sustaining and massive.

Qualities of Earth: Earth is cold and dry and very slow moving. It is mountains, rocks, the soil, our physical world. Earth governs the vegetable kingdom and the mineral kingdom and humankind. Earth rules the skeletal system, the body, flesh, matter and stuff. Earth measures both time and timelessness; it embodies endurance, patience, depth, permanence, growth and nourishment. Conversely, it can suffocate and restrict movement, slow down and block. It is protectionist and puts up walls and barriers.

Physical Earth: is in touch with the physical senses; the here and now reality of the material world. Earth feels rather than reasons (Air), senses (Water), or is inspired (Fire). Earth is attuned to the world of form and represents patience, self-discipline, continuing until the job is done, endurance, caution, convention; it is dependable, pre-meditative and acquisitive. Distrustful of the speed and noise of Air and Fire, Earth has an affinity with Water's self-protectiveness and both Water and Earth dislike change and letting go.

Psychological Earth: Jung gives Earth to sensation types, who understand their world through the five senses, seeing, hearing, tasting, smell, and touch. They distrust any information that does not come in this form. Earth finds fulfilment in service, practical helping. Its practicality is regardless of logic or feeling or inspiration. Earth moves slowly, like the mountains, crushing opposition, rarely roused to anger. Earth, once enraged, is as implacable and deadly as an earthquake. Ashes to ashes, dust to dust, Earth respects the physicality and structure of the human form and is only concerned with that; philosophical musings, speed, theories, psychic impressions, and feelings are anathema to Earth, which wants evidence it can see, touch, feel and smell. Stones are Earth's most durable manifestation; they are used as altars and houses, built up as sacred space. Earth's power lies in resilience and passivity.

It lacks the thinking of Air, the feeling of Water and the enterprise of Fire but gives us protection, safety, boundaries, and abundant fertility. Earth is responsible, reliable, thoughtful, courteous, mature and kind.

Emotional Earth: Earth is slow to warm to people but also loyal and dependable. Deeply suspicious, Earth distrusts noise, brightness, and ideas which come out of nowhere. Earth likes routine, the predictable, that which can be measured and nailed down. So, change is shocking, unsettling, disturbing, and Earth resists, hoards, and rejects the new. Earth's fear, unlike Water's, is deep and dark and terrifying and may cause her to be cruel and suffocating in order to feel safe. But she is dependable and reliable and diligent and offers practical solutions to problems. Earth is grounded and understands limits and time, and the need for preparation and order. Earth likes companionship to share the good things in life; food, nature, sex, all the pleasures of the senses. Earth can be a bit suffocating as they prefer to stay close, are unhurried and measured, but they are reliable and responsible. Slow to react, Earth has a fearsome temper: think landslides, the power of falling rock, earthquakes, the movement of glaciers over thousands of years. Because of its constancy and serious sense of commitment, Earth is predisposed to obsessions and ruminating, can become bitter, holding on too long; resentment is a live issue for Earth types. Cold and dry, Earth is inclined to depression. Sinking and slowing down come naturally and they can slip into deep, negative moods. They are susceptible to obsessive compulsive diseases, where the mind becomes fixed in a loop of intrusive thoughts and the anxiety is allayed by touching, counting, and other ritualised behaviour. Conversely, although they tend to bottle up uncomfortable emotions, when their anger does break out it can be earth-shattering and destructive. Cornered, Earth will charge like a rhinoceros and not stop until their enemy is destroyed, but they are not so much vindictive and cruel (as Fire is) but terrified, and their crushing of opponents is to deal with the source of pain once and for all.

Negative Earth: is slow, stubborn, unimaginative, dull-witted, very pessimistic and fearful. They may prefer animals to people, as they find emotions baffling and uninteresting. Some accuse them of being dull and boring, their love of routine and predictability can be exasperating. Emotionally they can be suspicious, resentful, bitter, grudge-bearers, mean and negative.

Lack of Earth: is spaced out, has difficulty negotiating the physical world, dislikes responsibility, is rootless, unable to support itself, has

survival issues. Lack of Earth shows a disregard and dislike of the physical body, is weak and flighty as they have no stamina or persistence.
They are flaky, unreliable, and may promise much but deliver little, can
be dishonest, shifty and unreliable.

Excess Earth: obsessive, mean, retentive, narrow-minded, suspicious.
They show a stolid dullness, have a lack of imagination, are dominated
by work and duty, lacking a sense of fun. They can be fixed, rigid and
lumpen. They are cynical and sceptical, mean, greedy, self-indulgent,
and judgemental.

Spirituality of Earth: Earth finds spiritual solace in the natural world,
among plants and animals, in nature and stones and crystals and big
trees and grains of sand. Earth will be attracted to silent, walking meditation, the spirituality of bhakti yoga—the yoga of service, washing the
feet of lepers, handing out soup to the homeless, building shelters for
the dispossessed. Without form we can do nothing in this life. Earth
understands this and respects and cares for her body and the body of
Gaia. Paracelsus gave Earth to gnomes who embody cheerfulness and
generosity. In Greek philosophy Earth represents the Dionysian nature;
Dionysus is the god of wine and dance, of sensuality, and the gratification of carnal desires, without logic or empathy.

Social Earth: Disliking change, Earth choses their companions care-
fully and then sticks to them. Earth prefers simple pleasures, a long
walk in the forest, a meal with friends, less interested in parties and
more in deep, soulful communication. Earth will be the friends who
help you dig your garden, or paint a room; uncomplicated, reliable,
trustworthy, not exciting perhaps, but steadfast and thoughtful.

Melancholic temperament

Physical characteristics

Like the element Earth, melancholic people and heavy, weighted, solid,
ponderous. They are not often obese, but they are solid, have a cart-
horse-like quality of putting their head down and plodding on. While
Fire is hot, Earth is cold; while Fire is dashing energy, Earth is building,
rootedness, calmness, and slowness. They do not like sudden movements, change, noise, or heat, but routine, predictability, and rhythm.
They have great stamina and are marathon runners rather than sprint-
ers, hill walkers and painstaking mountain climbers.

Emotional characteristics

Melancholics' chilliness extends to their emotions. They can be cold, cut off, and slow to react. Conservative, they value time, calmness, and predictability, and when faced with sudden upsets, change or noise, they can dig their heels in and refuse to budge. They smother the bright spark of fire with practicalities and doubts, for they are pessimistic and can be mean-spirited and avaricious. They do not trust the bright and shiny, but value tradition, painstaking work, slow ascents and careful planning. Depression can be a problem for a melancholic but their pessimism can bring happiness, or at least contentment, because they can often be pleasantly surprised when things work out. Their practicality works well with Fire's enthusiasm; Fire provides the inspiration and melancholics can work out the plan and execute the job in an orderly fashion.

In health

Generally, melancholics have a strong constitution and a heavy, dense, physical frame. Because cold slows things down, they suffer from poor digestion, slow metabolism, which can cause weight gain. They may find it hard to get going, unlike Fire, but once in motion it is difficult to stop or change direction. They may overwork and wear themselves down physically due to their doggedness to finish the job.

In sickness

Due to their coldness, melancholics may suffer from conditions of retention and blockages, slowness and stagnation. Cold and dryness can cause things to get stuck, frozen, impacted and ossified, and shows in sickness such as stones, bony overgrowths, tumours, and hard swellings. Melancholics have strength but low vitality and may suffer from overwork or low mood and depression. Melancholy is the temperament of old age, and they do indeed grow in strength and confidence as they get older, although they are often awkward and lonely children.

Regimen for melancholy

Melancholy has a poor digestion and so should eat very sparingly and lightly, non-greasy food such as grains. They should avoid cold foods unless they live in a warm climate. They also should rest enough to avoid burnout, but not so much that they cannot get going again. Time spent in nature is healing and restoring to the melancholic, so suggest to them activities like gardening and walking. They respond to ritual and routine, so exercise can be factored in to their daily activities and, once the habit is acquired, they will keep doing it. Pastimes can be used to explore unexpressed elements; in the case of melancholy, adventure, romance, intellectual exploration, and rest will help to counter their attachment to routine.

Culpeper on melancholy abounding

They suffer from fearfulness without cause, fearful and foolish imaginations. Their skin is rough and swarthy. They are lean and bony. They can suffer from poor sleep and frightful dreams. Their pulse is weak, the urine thin and clear. They are often loners and may sigh as they speak. (Culpeper, 1653, p. 88.)

Culpeper continues:

A Melancholly person is one whose Body cold and driness is predominate, and not such a one as is sad somtimes as the vulgar dream, they are usually slender and not very tall, of swarthy duskish colour, rough Skin, cold and hard in feeling, they have very little Hair on their Bodies and are long without Beards, and somtimes they are Beardless in age, the Hair of their Heads is dusky brown usually, and somtimes duskie flaxen their appetite is far better than their concoction usually, by reason appetite is caused of a sowr vapor sent up by the Spleen which is the Seat of Melancholly, to the Stomach, their Urine is pale, their dung of a clayish colour and broken, their Pulse slow, they dream of frightful things, black, darkness, and terrible businesses. (Culpeper, 1653, p. 62.)

They are naturally Covetous, Self-lovers, Cowards, afraid of their own Shadows, fearful, careful, solitary, lumpish, unsociable, delighting to be alone, stubborn, ambitious, Envious, of a deep cogitation, obstinate in Opinion, mistrustful, suspicious, spiteful, squemish, and yet slovenly, they retain Anger long, and aim at no smal things. (Culpeper, 1652, p. 55.)

Diet and exercise fitting

> [L]et Melancholly Men avoid excess both in eating and drinking, let them avoid all meats hard of digestion, especially such as are Students or lead a Sedentary life; let them use meats that are light of digestion, and drink often at meat. Excess either in meat or strong liquor, causeth crudities and rawness at the Stomach, Idle and strange imaginatious and fancies, a stinking Breath, Headach, Toothach, forgetfulness, shortness of breath, Consumptions, Phtisicks, third day Agues, the Chollick and Illiack passions, and Dropsies.
>
> Much Exercise is very profitable for such, not only because it helpeth digestion, but also, because it destributeth the Vital Spirit throughout the Body, and consumeth those superfluous Vapors by insensible Transpiration, which causeth those idle fancies and imaginations in men. (Culpeper, 1652, p. 54.)

The Earth signs ♉ ♍ ♑

Taurus ♉

Nature

Taurus is cold, dry, earthy, melancholy, feminine, fixed (because when the Sun moves into these signs the season, in this case spring, is fixed), and ruled by Venus. Taurus is vernal or a spring sign (like Aries and Gemini). The Moon is exalted in Taurus and Mars is in detriment. Taurus rules the throat.

Famous Taureans

Charlotte Bronte, William Shakespeare, Queen Elizabeth II.

Physical

As an Earth sign, Taurus usually has a strong, solid body, not tall, but thickset and hardworking. Ruled by Venus they are often attractive, sensual, rounded, and feminine or softly masculine. They often have large, soulful eyes—cow-like—and lustrous hair. They move slowly, with dignity, and present an unruffled demeanour. Fairly silent, Taurus watches and weighs things up before speaking, not from shyness but because she is calmly appraising the situation and making a judgement about what her reaction should be. Often, they have a pleasant, soft voice.

Emotional

Taurus, as an Earth sign, dislikes noise and excitement; she prefers order and calm and dignity. Her serene appearance is deceptive, however. Slow to anger, when she does lose her temper her rage is formidable and terrifying, like a raging bull, and will continue until her adversary is crushed underfoot. A lover of beauty and nature, many artists and musicians are found in this sign as it has the sensual and artistic appreciation together with practical skills and the capacity for hard work. Once Taurus gets going she continues until the end, and it is hard to move her off-track. Stubborn to the point of insensibility, Taurus does not change her mind much and likes routine and predictability. Her love of beauty can make her acquisitive and greedy. She shows affection through the material world, gifts, and food principally, but love and relationships are very important to her, expressed practically and sensually, with loyalty and steadfastness.

Mental

Because of her stubbornness, Taurus is prone to obsessions and compulsions as she will not let go of an idea. Change is difficult, and Taurus can get stuck in a rut, physically, emotionally, and mentally. Her materialism can cause depression, due to spending beyond her means or the realisation that material things will not make her safe or loved. Nature is a great source of pleasure and can provide solace and healing for Taurus.

Illnesses

All diseases of the throat, tonsillitis, quinsy, hoarseness. Due to her love of food, obesity and its resulting problems can be an issue. All the Earth signs are prone to depression, being melancholic, cold, and dry, they find it hard to deal with their emotions and tend to be pessimistic and gloomy, or rigid and unyielding. Culpeper writes: "Under Taurus all diseases incident to the throat, as Kings evill, quinsy, soare throat, wenns in the neck, flux of rheume in the throat" (Culpeper, 1651a, p. 90).

Cures

If the physician or the medicine is shown by planets in Taurus, use herbs, massage, aromatherapy, any touch-based therapy, and also creative therapies, such as art therapy and dance therapy. Encourage exercise to get the energy moving, gentle yoga, dance, tai chi, gardening, or walking. For Taurus suggest a clean diet low on carbs, but not cold food (salads or dairy). Taurus can be chilly and stagnant; gently warming drinks and foods with ginger are recommended. Avoid sugar; Taurus has a great sweet tooth and is prone to candida, diabetes, and obesity.

Virgo ♍

Nature

Virgo is an Earth sign, cold and dry, melancholic, feminine, and mutable (Lilly calls this "common" [Lilly, 1647, p. 88]) that is, they have some of the properties of the preceding sign and the following sign. Other mutable signs are Gemini, Sagittarius, and Pisces. Lilly considers people shown by mutable signs neither "willful" (cardinal) nor fixed (Lilly, 1647, p. 89).

Famous Virgos

Queen Elizabeth I, Michael Jackson, Agatha Christie.

Dignity and debility

Virgo is the house and exaltation of Mercury. Jupiter is in detriment in Virgo and Venus is in fall. Virgo is a barren sign, showing few or no children. Virgo is one of the humane or courteous signs; if these signs ascend or the Lord of the Ascendant is in these signs, the man will be "of civil carriage, very affable and easie to be spoken withall" (Lilly, 1647, p. 89).

Physical

Virgo, like Gemini (which is also ruled by Mercury), gives a slight, androgynous, youthful body and demeanour. They will be slight, restless, and often have small hands and feet, ageless faces, and a pixie-like quality. Virgo rules the gut (the Moon rules the stomach) and, being ruled by Mercury, the nervous system. Lilly describes Virgo as having: "a slender body of meane height, but decently composed … a small shrill voice, all members inclining to brevity; a witty discreet soul, judicious and excellently well spoken [Mercury], studious, given to history, whether man or woman it produceth a rare understanding … but somewhat unstable" (Lilly, 1647, p. 96).

Emotional

Virgo is full of nervous energy and this can be expressed as either a perfectionist or a chaotic hoarder. Virgo finds life's confusion difficult to negotiate and tries to think its way out of emotional distress, which naturally is a difficult proposition, as emotions are neither logical nor orderly. Virgo can be very wound up and they often somaticize anxiety, which in turn increases tension in the body, creating a vicious cycle of stress and anxiety. Look for emotional causes in diseases shown by Virgo. Like Capricorn, Virgo has a predisposition to obsessive compulsive conditions, especially phobias around dirt and hygiene.

Mental

Virgos are gentle, thoughtful, and considerate people, who distrust speedy, flashy, noisy types. They ponder deeply and worry at problems, but may lack the self-confidence to express themselves. They have a grace and elegance which is unshowy. Again, overthinking is an issue here: they are great organisers and systematisers, but apart from filing systems, and pure science, there is little in life that can be organised so logically. Like Taurus, Virgo can be prone to depression, being of a generally pessimistic disposition with the added extra of anxiety. Mind control is key here.

Illnesses

Virgo often presents with emotional gut problems, such as cramp, wind, diarrhoea, or more serious diseases of the intestines such as leaky gut (allergies), diverticulitis, Crohn's disease, etc. Lilly writes: "winde, collicke, all obstructions in the bowels … croking of the Guts … any disease of the belly" (Lilly, 1647, p. 96). There is often a strong, stressful component to any illness; Virgo can sometimes be described as the astrological sign of psychosomatic illness. Culpeper describes "hardening of the spleen" in Virgo; the spleen is "the seat of the melancholic humour and associated with the retentive virtue" (Culpeper, 1651a, p. 91). All the Earth signs, being cold and dry, are prone to blockage (retention). "Hypochondriac melancholy" arises, the *hupokhondrion* being the abdominal area beneath the breastbone, including the spleen, which the Greeks gave as the seat of the melancholy humour; hypochondria, then, is an illness of the gut brought on by melancholy rather than an imaginary illness (Houlding, 2007).

Treatments

If I had my way, all Virgos would be taught yoga and meditation from a very young age, which would free up their mental faculties for positive ends. Virgo shows a need to re-direct worry from their bodies to problem-solving elsewhere. Their digestion is not great at the best of times, and so an allergy diet (gluten-free, dairy-free, additive-free) is ideal, together with some form of exercise that can calm the mind. Insomnia can be an issue, as the Virgo mind finds it hard to turn off, in which case gentle, herbal relaxants will help.

Capricorn ♑

Nature

Melancholic, cold, dry, cardinal, ruled by Saturn, Mars is exalted in Capricorn, the Moon is in detriment, and Jupiter is in fall.

Famous Capricorns

Martin Luther King, Joseph Stalin, Stephen Hawking, Simon Wiesenthal.

Dignity and debility

Capricorn rules the winter, old age, the winter solstice.

Physical

Capricorn rules the knees, bones in general, the teeth, the ears. Their bodies are dry and sparse, bony, hairy, dark or swarthy, and plain-looking. Capricorns look older than their years, with a serious expression, and are often stooping and clumsy.

Emotional

Capricorn is serious and can be gloomy and pessimistic. Very ambitious, patient, and calculating they often rise to the top of their career due to their persistence, dedication, and hard work. Often highly intelligent, they can be emotionally cold and critical to those who do not live up to their high standards. Old before their time, they are conventional and fearful of dishonour, which can make them timid or causes them to hold back until later in life when experience has given them the confidence to speak out. Suspicious of the motives of others, they are often lonely as teenagers and young people, being overly serious and staid.

Mental

Known for their logical powers of deliberation, Capricorns are studious and intelligent. Like the other Earth signs they are prone to negative thinking and depression. Capricorn, ruled by Saturn, has a reputation for being gloomy and pessimistic and struggles with morbid fear and fantasies. They often feel misunderstood, especially when young, and can be isolated and unpopular. Things improve with time, though, and Capricorn excels in middle and old age.

Illnesses

Diseases of the bones such as osteoarthritis and rheumatism, fractures, broken bones, pulled ligaments and tendons. Culpeper says: "Under Capricorne are all diseases in the knees and hams; as pains, sprains, fractures, and dislocations, leprosies, itch, scabs, all diseases of melancholie" (Culpeper, 1651a, p. 93). Being cold and dry, Capricorn rules stones, blockages, or hard swellings, deafness and tooth decay. The ugly side of Capricorn rules disfiguring skin diseases, such as psoriasis and scabies, hirsutism, and any birth defect that affects the appearance. Depression is another condition found in Capricorn.

Treatment

Time in nature is always healing for Capricorn. Gardening is a good way to connect with the earth and slowly work on a project to relax. Bodywork would be good, although it is not much liked by this stiff, inflexible sign. Capricorn prefers exclusion diets, lots of structure in their treatment, and a good rationale or explanation for your treatment plan. They need to feel confidence in your expertise, so your professionalism and qualifications will be important to them.

Water

Water meditation

Deep lake, dark water, you are held on its silky surface, buoyantly floating. The ancient waters drag you down. Slowly you sink weightless in the darkness. The water holds you and pulls you inwards. You slip deeper. Flashes of light illuminate brightly-coloured fish. Their blind eyes turn towards you, sensing movement, a disturbance in the stillness. Figures dive and twist out of caves, wraith-like, transparent, long tendrils of seaweed twist and bob behind them. They take you by the hand. There are more of them, and more again. In a crowd you are pulled into deeper and darker water. Fear flies across your heart. All the shapes are mysterious, distorted. Your breath becomes laboured as your chest is crushed by the weight of the water. In a gasp, you are on the surface again. Sunlight dapples the surface of the water, shooting rainbows of light across the surface. Light, warm rain begins to fall. You swim on, cresting the shallow waves, which deepen and grow, the wavelets becoming waves and then breakers. You are flung and tossed and bounce and dive on the sheer wall of water. You feel exhilaration, and weightlessness. Then the waves pound the shore. They spit you out as they roar and crash around you, sucking in trees and buildings and tiny boats, which are swallowed by the whirlpool. The ferocity and power of the water is terrifying. On the beach you land near a small tributary and lean over, drinking the sweet water. It is like nectar; sooth-ing, refreshing, healing. Water.

Water is cold and wet. It has the qualities of change, flux, move-ment, great power, gentle change. It dissolves and over time can wear away the highest cliffs. Earth can overcome Water, by filling in a pond, for example, whereas Water can break down Earth by erosion or tidal waves. We are aquatic creatures; we came from water onto dry land. As developing embryos we have gills. Our lungs do not operate until we are in the air; we float in fluid in the womb. We are watery. Power-ful as a tidal wave and as delicate as morning dew, Water holds the earth together, giving moist soil a malleability and cohesiveness. When Earth lacks Water, it blows away as dust. Too much Water dissolves and disperses Earth, turning the fixed and dense into slippery, liquid mud. Water has a sinking, heavy quality. It fills all the available space, equal-ising and finding its own level.

Water has magical properties. Recognising the urgent human need for water, wells are dressed, sacred springs are worshipped, and under-ground water courses can be divined by a hazel rod. The deep well is a metaphor for how we inquire into spirit; do we skim the surface or haul secrets from the dark, deep source?[1] Holy water blesses, protects, renews, cleanses, re-births, the dead are washed, the holy are anointed, we wash our hands and feet to cleanse our souls. The moon pulls the tides and draws blood from our watery bodies and on occasion raises our sensitivity to bursting.

Keywords for Water: Cold. Wet. Heavy. Sinking. Flooding. Moisten-ing. Softening. Diluting. Adaptable. Changeable. Dissolving.

Water almost combines the other elements: it has the quality of no fixed shape, like Air, and takes on the colour of its surroundings; it has the stability and endurance of Earth; and its effortlessness is like fire. Water provides the source of inspiration; unlike Air, which is rational thought, the wisdom of water bubbles up from a deep, unknown, hid-den place of knowing and wisdom, the stream of consciousness. Water is not linear and defined but takes the shape of the container within which it is placed: tears, rivers, raindrops, oceans, mist, ice. Water is the imagination and is indirect, elusive, unfathomable. It provides the

---

[1]See for example the *I Ching*, hexagram 48: *Ching*, the Well.

profundities of spiritual experience rather than the dogma of religion, which may be earthy or airy.

Water is both formless and unifying. With Water, there is no chaos or fragmentation; on the contrary, Water unites and connects. The oceans connect continents, and rivers connect the interior with the outside world, mountains with the beach. It is seamless and cannot be broken, but it can be transformed, to ice, mist, vapour, and back again. Water cannot lose its fundamental nature and always has the potential to return to its original state. O'Donohue talks of the indifference of Water; put a finger into a glass of water and then remove it, no difference has been made (O'Donohue, 2007, p. 47). Water flows until it finds its level and travels downhill, taking the easiest route to equilibrium. Oceans have no marker; sailors use the stars to plot their course, because Water cannot be mapped, it is too inconstant. Spring rains bring growth, green shoots, summer flowers; they revitalise the earth and cleanse the air.

Lack of water: leads to hardness, dryness, barrenness, inflexibility, stuck-ness, blockages.

Psychology of Water: Water represents the astral body, dominated by yearnings. It has the Dionysian quality of desires, feelings, unconscious and instinctual forces. Water shows creativity, nuances, subtleties, fears, love and acceptance. Water can be motivated by the unconscious mind and be unaware of what drives it. Watery types are psychically sensitive, empathetic, and responsive to people. When they are not aware they can be compulsive, hyper-sensitive and have irrational fears. As Water has no form, watery types are happiest when they are channelled by other people and given a structure. Water mixes especially well with Earth, which provides boundaries and calm. They dislike the noisy and strident Air and Fire people, preferring security and self-protection. Water is secretive and self-contained; the storms of emotion which rage beneath the surface can cause them to explode dramatically. Water also creates emotional storms and dramas if bored or ignored. Water has great sensitivity, but also great power. Water conquers by yielding and slowly dissolving opposition; they can be implacable, wearing down the other elements by manipulation or "soft power". Highly impressionable, Water needs solitude to wash away other people's energies and recharge themselves. They long to be close to the sea. Paracelsus' assignment of spirits to elements gives undines to Water, which can only be controlled by firmness.

Physical Water: Water in the body lubricates, softens, mixes, discharges. It causes bloating, fluid retention, coldness, slowness, dullness, constant pain, excessive sleeping, lethargy, low energy, debility. Physically, Water shows up as menstrual issues, reproductive issues, cold diseases, wet diseases, physical conditions with emotional causes, vomiting, diarrhoea.

Positive Water: Water is empathetic, kind, gentle, caring, perceptive, creative, unifying, peaceful, attractive, harmonious, resilient, adaptable, persistent, forgiving, and beautiful.

Negative Water: Is fearful, lazy, passive, dependent, greedy, manipulative, negative, pessimistic, and clingy.

Lack of Water: This shows a person lacking in empathy, callous and aloof, who will disregard, dismiss and ridicule the feelings of others. They deny their emotional nature and vulnerabilities, which often makes them unconsciously dependent on people who are in contact with their feelings. They are lonely, disconnected from others, unsympathetic and harsh. They can project their unacknowledged feelings, attacking the openness of those persons they project upon, or be emotionally toxic, full of denied emotional baggage expressed as hostility and coldness.

Excess Water: This shows people who are easily influenced, often lacking direction and willpower. Water overreacts emotionally, can feel haunted, prone to sulking, or may use extreme behaviour to manipulate others. Their self-sacrifice may be genuine or mask absolute selfishness and their need to control through emotional blackmail and drama.

Spiritual Water: Water produces the mystics, who long for union with the divine, who gain spiritual insights through dreams, meditation, and psychic messages. Strong Water is found in intuitive painters, musicians, dancers, mediums who talk with other worlds. Water can express deep empathy and compassion for suffering.

Phlegmatic temperament

Physical characteristics

Cold and wet, the phlegmatic type has the biggest body and can run to obesity in later life. They suffer from water retention; their skin is cold and clammy. They feel the cold but hate to move around;

exercise is anathema to them. They are slow-moving, often lethargic, sleep a lot, like to comfort-eat, and prefer home and safety and security. Generally, they are hairless or have thin hair and are pale and pasty.

Emotional characteristics

Phlegmatics *feel*. Their emotional lives are rich and profound, but they can find the hard edges of "ordinary" life painful to deal with. They are prone to fear and their morbid ruminations can overtake their lives with anxiety, insomnia, and phobias. Conversely, their great sensitivity makes them psychic, spiritual, compassionate, and loving. Because of the slowness they embody, they can become trapped in negative states and need a bit of Fire to overcome them. To soften life's hard edges, they sometimes self-medicate with alcohol and drugs, or bliss out on meditation, music, food, dance, or even television.

In health

Although emotionally volatile, physically the phlegmatic can show surprising resilience, as Water is adaptable and mutable. In patients, psychosomatic illnesses need to be considered as their emotional response is so strong. Keeping the emotions clear and moving will preserve their health.

In sickness

Fluid and fears are the main expressions of a phlegmatic. They suffer from coughs with phlegm, discharges (such as heavy periods, diarrhoea, suppurating wounds), oedema, swellings, coldness, dull pains which linger, palpitations, anxiety, insomnia. Phlegmatics are prone to night terrors, hauntings, panic attacks, and anxiety. Addictions, lethargy, obesity, coldness, are all phlegmatic diseases.

Regimen for phlegmatic

Because their boundaries are a bit porous, phlegmatics need to learn to protect and ground themselves. They need to eat the least amount of food (but are the most likely to want to comfort-eat) and they need to sleep the minimum number of hours (although they love to hide in bed). Exercise is great for them, but it is a challenge to persuade them to do it; suggest dancing, tai chi, yin yoga (the movements of which are slow and graceful). They do not tolerate—but often take—alcohol and recreational drugs to dull their sensitivities. They would be better learning meditation and psychic protection and earthing techniques, as they are more sensitive than the other temperaments, and substance abuse is a real issue for them.

Culpeper on the phlegmatic temperament

[… T]hey are very dull, heavy and slothful, like the Scholler that was a great while a learning a Lesson, but when Once he had it—he had quickly forgotten it: They are drowsie, sleepy, cowardly forgetful Creatures, as swift in motion as a Snail, they travail (and that's but seldom) as though they intended to go 15. miles in 14. daies, yet are they shame fac'd and sober.

People of this Complexion of all other ought to use a very slender Diet, for fasting clenseth the Body of those gross and unconcocted Humors which Flegmatick People are usually as full of as an Egg is of Meat: What they do eat, let it be of light digestion, a Cup of strong Beer, and now and then a cup of Wine is no waies unwholsom for them of this Complexion that are minded to keep their Bodies in health. Much Meat and Drink fills their Bodies full of Indigestion, Wind, and Stitches, Quotidian Agues and Dropsies, Falling sickness and Gouts, Rhewms and Catharres. Much Exercise is very healthful for them unless they love their laziness better than their health, for by that means gross Humors are made thin and expelled by sweat, the Memory is quickned and the Skin clarified. (Culpeper, 1652, p. 56.)

Culpeper on signs of phlegm abounding

Shows sleepiness, dullness, heaviness, slowness, cowardliness, forgetfulness, much spitting, much superfluities at the nose, little appetite, bad digestion, white skin, cold and hairless, urine thick and pale, dreams of rain, floods etc. (Culpeper, 1653, p. 62.)

The Water signs ♋ ♏ ♓

Cancer ♋

Nature

Cancer is cardinal water, cold, moist, phlegmatic, feminine, ruled by the Moon only, the sign of the summer solstice, fertile,[2] and mute.[3] It shows winter (along with the other phlegmatic signs).

Famous Cancerians

Nelson Mandela, the Duke of Windsor, Meryl Streep, Elizabeth Kübler Ross (see below for a discussion of her chart).

Dignity and debility

Jupiter is exalted in Cancer, Saturn is in detriment, and Mars is in fall.

Physical

Generally, Water signs have a softness about them, reflecting their watery nature. Some may have the classic "moon face", round like the full moon, and often they have soft, sweet voices and are attractive in a gentle, motherly way. They can become fat due to water retention, and are rarely bony, but often soft-looking. They often have big, soulful, deep eyes, and a hesitancy or guardedness on first meeting. Low energy and lassitude are Cancerian traits, especially at full and new moon. They like to move slowly and hate noise and bustle. Cancer rules the stomach, the breasts, and the water balance in the body.

Emotional

The sign of the mother, Cancer has a soft, maternal character, and both men and women will be very attached to home and partners. They

---

[2]The other fertile signs are Scorpio and Pisces (Lilly, 1647, p. 89).
[3]Or "of slow voice". Other mute signs are Scorpio and Pisces (Lilly, 1647, p. 89). Einstein was considered to be "subnormal" because he did not speak until aged three and not fluently until aged nine. Yet, by age thirteen, he had read Euclid's *Geometry* and the rest, as we say, is history. Einstein had the Sun and midheaven in Pisces and ascendant in Cancer. It might be argued that he didn't speak because he was communicating in ways other than those usually open to an infant.

are clannish and draw friends close and banish outsiders. Cancer *feels*; sometimes the intensity of their emotions can be overwhelming. They are changeable (like the Moon), moody, can be over-sensitive and hysterical, or brooding and fearful. However, as we discussed with regard to the element Water, Cancerians have great strength and fortitude and can weather many storms due to their adaptability and changeable nature; flexibility gives them strength. They can be insensitive to other people's feelings, more concerned to "circle the waggons" rather than offer a helping hand.

Mental

Prone to fears and worrying, Cancer can get lost in indecision and mental confusion. However, their deep well of wisdom can often surprise. Never one for a quick opinion, Cancer, by musing on problems, often bring to the surface bright pearls of wisdom other signs miss through hurry or lack of imagination. They are inherently creative; many writers are Cancerians because they can work at home (Cancer's favourite place) and sit in solitude with their imagination, dreaming up new worlds. They are reflective like the Moon, and can take on their surroundings, or adapt to their company.

Illnesses

Cancer shows stomach complaints like cramp, and pains which may be due to anxiety or "undigested emotions" affecting the stomach. Classic Cancer is gut ache and diarrhoea before a big event. Their phlegmatic nature gives them a weak digestion, but despite this they may overeat and suffer from weight gain, gastric reflux and bloating. Swelling due to water retention is seen and cold (white) discharges, such as excess phlegm in coughs and leucorrhoea. Lilly gives Cancer to "Cancers which are ever in the breast" (Lilly, 1647, p. 95). Culpeper adds, "whatsoever are incident to the breasts of women … inflamation, which women commonly call the imposthumes [abscesses, also mastitis], want of appetite to victuals, want of digestion of Victuals, coldnesse and over-heat of the stomack, dropsies, coughes; you may find out the rest your selves; the rule is as plaine as the nose in a man's face" (Culpeper, 1651a, p. 90).

Because of their powerful emotions, consider an emotional root cause if the sickness is shown by Cancer, and treat their feelings as well as any physical symptoms.

Treatment

Cancer wants comfort above all else. A disease shown by Cancer shows the need for gentle, nourishing remedies, which build up stamina and put a bit of fire in the belly. They will resist exercise, so suggest dance or gentle massages to bring them back in their bodies. Symptoms will wax and wane as the Moon does, so it is important to keep firmly to a treatment plan despite fluctuations. Cancer is prone to anxiety and phobias: Bach flower remedies or herbal remedies for the nervous system are very helpful. Avoid any heroic treatments, high doses, or strong remedies; they will react strongly and negatively.

Scorpio ♏

Nature

Scorpio is fixed water, phlegmatic, cold and moist, feminine, the autumn, a mute sign and fruitful.

Famous Scorpios

Pablo Picasso, Bill Gates, Hilary Clinton, Nicholas Culpeper.

Dignity and debility

Scorpio is ruled by Mars, traditionally, and latterly Pluto. The Moon is in fall and Venus in detriment in the sign.

Physical

One trait all Scorpios share is their disconcerting, piercing gaze. They have an animal magnetism and virility which is potent and bold. Like Cancer, Scorpio has a soft body and round face, but behind this is the burning energy and dynamism of Mars. Restless, brooding, disconcerting, they do not put people at ease like Cancer, rather, they provoke and challenge, but in a watery, roundabout way. Physically strong, Scorpio can use will-power alone to surmount physical limitations. Lilly describes Scorpio: "somehwat bow-legged, short necked, a squat, wel-trussed fellow'" (Lilly, 1647, p. 97). Scorpio rules the genitals, the bladder and anus, sexual potency, and fertility in men and women.

Emotional

Deep, Scorpio inhabits the darkest places of the psyche and there is nothing about human nature that surprises or disappoints. If you want to know what is happening, ask a Scorpio, their watchful, psychic antennae understand the most buried, unconscious motives behind people's behaviour. They love danger, physical or emotional, and will push boundaries to the extreme, and then some. Their Machiavellian drives can backfire, and they take failure hard and very, very personally, holding grudges for decades while plotting revenge. Emotional poisoning then, is often an issue; toxic thoughts, jealousy, envy, ambition, power struggles, revenge are all in Scorpio's domain. Conversely, their perception, forensic and penetrating, cannot be bettered. As Lilly puts it, "usually it doth represent subtill, deceitful men" (Lilly, 1647, p. 97).

Mental

Extreme and sometimes pathological competitiveness is a Scorpio trait. They would see this as a compliment, because why would you wish to be other than the richest, most powerful, or sexually attractive? Second place is losing. They are driven and can use underhand and downright dishonest tactics to succeed, but, generally, succeed they will. Focus, mental acuity, and foresight ensure that Scorpio will reach their goal. Because of this Scorpio tends to attract enemies, both real and imagined, which may give rise to paranoia, pre-emptive strikes, cruelty, isolation, and mental breakdown.

Illnesses

Poisoning is the word for Scorpio. Physically, illness from infection, such as STDs, AIDS, boils, septicaemia, any poisoning from food, chemicals, or the environment. Also, diseases of the genitalia and bladder; any condition with pus and infection throughout the body; fistulae and haemorrhoids and womb infections with noxious discharges, and pain such as pelvic inflammatory disease, or bacterial vaginosis. Emotional poisoning in the form of paranoia or psychosis can come under Scorpio. Culpeper says: "Under the Scorpion are gravell and stone in the bladder, inflammations and ulcers there, all difficulties of urine whatsoever; all imperfections of the urine, ruptures, fistulaes, hemorrhoids, the french pox, running of the reines, priapismus; all diseases that infect the privities of men or women, All diseases of the wombe" (Culpeper, 1651a, p. 93).

Treatment

Again, like Cancer it is important to treat underlying emotional issues when a disease is shown by Scorpio. Psychotherapy and hypnotherapy may be helpful, also meditation can help. Physically, strong remedies which purify the blood and the liver and kidneys are called for. Bach flower remedies may help release some emotional states. Tact is needed as Scorpio hates admitting weakness and vulnerability. A competitive physical discipline will appeal, such as ashtanga yoga or squash, and will help to keep the energy moving.

Pisces ♓

Nature

Mutable water, Pisces is phlegmatic, cold and moist, feminine, mute, fertile.

Famous Pisceans

Albert Einstein, Copernicus, Elizabeth Taylor, Roberto Assagioli.

Dignity and debility

Pisces is ruled by Jupiter and, since its discovery, Neptune. Venus is exalted in Pisces. Mercury is in detriment and fall.

Physical

The most languid of signs, Pisces does not have a great deal of energy, but it has great tenacity like all the Water signs. Pisces often gives great beauty. Pisces rules the feet, and perhaps the lymphatic system. Prone to water retention, Pisces can become obese; they are slow moving, placid, and sleepy. Pisces prefers the life of the imagination to the crude realities of the world. Lilly is not a fan: "an idle, effeminate, sickly sign" (Lilly, 1647, p. 99).

Emotional

Psychic, spiritual, haunted, clairvoyant, visionary, a dreamer, imaginative, escapist, manipulative, and compassionate, Pisces is like the wide ocean, carrying all manner of treasures and flotsam and jetsam in its depths. It is the sign of pioneers and visionaries, as well as drunkards and junkies. Pisces likes to escape the dreary everyday world and dream up pleasant futures. It may do this by examining the burning questions of spirituality, science or philosophy, or by self-medicating with drink and drugs. Prone to phobias and hauntings, they may use these psychic phenomena to interpret the world for clients, or they may become paralysed with fear and a little mad.

Mental

Although traditionally a sign of low intelligence, nevertheless scientists and philosophers and deep thinkers of all stripes are found in Pisces. Their unbounded imagination ranges far and wide, deep and high, and can penetrate the deepest mysteries. Conversely, they can be idle, loutish, and dumb; it depends if they rise to the challenge their perception offers them, or slump into safety, numbness, and anaesthesia. Their boundaries are weak, and they can feel invaded and controlled by others' thoughts.

Illnesses

Pisces shows any diseases of the feet, such as gout; cold and moist diseases, discharge, phlegm, rotten coughs, sinusitis; also, "corrupted blood", colds, boils, ulcers, and any swelling due to water retention. Culpeper adds:

> Under Pisces is all lamenesse, aches and diseases incident to the feet, as gouts, kibes [ulcerated chilblain], childblains, &c. All diseases coming of salt flegme, mixt humours, scabs, itch, botches, and breakings out about the body, the small poxe and measles; all cold and moist diseases, and such as come by catching wett and cold at the feet.
>
> And if you will be pleased but to consider the affinity Pisces holds with Aries, you will soon see a reason, why wet taken at the

feet strikes so speedily up to the head. As for the houses of the heavens, they have the same significations with the signs; the first house with Aries, the second with Taurus, and so analogically till you come to the twelfth house, which hath the same significations that Pisces hath. (Culpeper, 1651a, p. 94.)

Treatment

Use hot and drying herbs for phlegmatic illness, reduce the diet, avoid dairy products, sugar and grains, all of which increase Phlegm. Encourage exercise such as dancing, swimming, and discourage rest, over-sleeping and sedentary lifestyles. Use Bach flower remedies or other emotional-based practices for calming the emotions.

Air

Air meditation

Imagine you are floating in the warm air. Your body is weightless, held up by warm air currents. You move above the earth and the sea and the fire. Feel the air all around you. Breathe in the air and allow it to fill your body. Notice how your body feels, the speed you are moving at (if you are moving), how it feels to be in the air, held yet at the same time weightless. Feel the air in your organs. Notice any sensations or images which come up for you. Focus on your feelings; are there any emotions that come up, or images, or memories? Notice them and let them go. Be aware of your thoughts. Watch them as they pass by. Register them and then release them. The breeze carries you gently down to earth. Open your eyes and write down what happened.

Air is space, empty and full at the same time. We take our first breath; a huge intake expands the lungs and we are separate and alive and autonomous. Maybe we cry, or maybe the rush of sweet air calms the panic of breathlessness and we relax. We take our last breath; a shudder or a rattle or a slow exhale, and we separate from our physical bodies and perhaps return to the place we left when we took our first breath. Breath is life. We cannot live for five minutes without breathing. The feeling of not "catching" your breath is panic-inducing, ask any asthmatic—that feeling of being one non-inhaled moment away from death is terrifying.

The ebb and flow of breath sustains life and sets the rhythm of life. Pranayama is the Vedic science of breathing, "evenness of breathing leads to healthy nerves and so to evenness of mind and temper'" (Iyengar, 1974, p. 43). Breathing consciously draws the focus of the mind inwards and calms the chattering thoughts. Breath used consciously can control pain, and calm panic, and bring equilibrium and peace to the panicked mind.

Air is the great equaliser. We all breathe the same air: man, animals and plants. We breathe in and transform those ancient gases created in the aftermath of the Big Bang that have been circulating and nourishing all life ever since then. O'Donohue (2010, p. 32) writes that air is the most welcoming of the elements. Earth resists letting things in; Water lets things in, but remains itself; Fire lets things in, and then destroys them; whereas Air lets things in, and will do no damage to them. Air is also terrifying in its nothingness. It is huge, undifferentiated space, which has no edge, no boundary, and extends and seeps in everywhere. Air is the medium through which sound travels, heard but not seen. Air is sea breezes on a sweltering day, the sound of song, hurricanes and windchimes, burning desert air, and freezing polar winds. In the body, Air represents breath, the lungs, thought, mental and psychological issues, speech and hearing.

The ancients saw Air, the heavens, and the sky-gods who lived there, as hard, implacable beings who could throw thunderbolts, hurricanes, and tornadoes. The upper air is the home of the gods; many spiritual traditions speak of bridges, rainbows, world trees, which connect the mundane world with the rarefied Air of spirit. Iris in Greek mythology was the goddess of the rainbow; she spanned this divide and brought messages of peace. Birds are also messengers of the gods; they are magical beings who float in the invisible air. *Pneuma* (πνευμα) is the Greek word for Air or divine knowledge or reason. Air is vital spirit or breath, that which unites, connects, and coordinates the four humours.

Wind unleashed is terrifying. There is little that can withstand the brutal force of hurricanes; not buildings, for sure. In the tropics the safest place to be in a hurricane is in the mangroves whose rootedness, not in the earth but in the air, whose flexibility and pliability allows them to duck and weave, bend and sway, as the rushing air sweeps by and the flood waters rise.

Air gives space and without space individuality is impossible. But empty space, dark space, is terrifying, a silence and emptiness which extends in all directions. Air is nothingness, which is the opposite of Earth's acquisitiveness. The message of Air is to be attached to nothing and everything simultaneously.

Air represents the ideas behind the veil of the physical world, "in the beginning was the word" (John 1: 1), but *logos*, "word" in Ancient Greek (λoγoς), can mean any of the following: discourse, argument, speech, story, oracle, principle, maxim, proverb, promise, order, command, proposal, agreement, decision, fable, thought, deliberation, opinion, argument, and value (Liddell & Scott, 1944, p. 416). Try substituting some of these translations to the creation of the world.[1] In the beginning was: the decision (by whom?), the thought (of whom?), the story (of what?), the argument (between who?), the promise (to whom?), the order (from whom?). The delight and dilemma of Air is revealed: endless options, neither good nor bad, positive nor negative, right nor wrong, unravel before us and on and on come the computations and alternatives. It is both exciting and exhausting. Earth, who likes to know where she is, despairs at Air's inconstancy and mutability. Unsubtle Fire dismisses the myriad of options and takes the first choice. Water cannot understand Air any more than Air appreciates Water; there is no common language.

Qualities of Air: Air represents the intellect, thought, the abstract mind, the mental body, the thought patterns of the Universal Mind. It rules forms of thought, theories, and concepts. Air is detached and lacks emotion; it is the abstract, the theoretical. In extremis Air can be cruel, fanatical, and eccentric. If Air's opinions or ideas are ignored or challenged it is threatened. Air is fulfilled by learning.

Physical Air: Air has trouble with physicality; it does not like the restraints and limitations of the physical body and the material world. Often Air has immature or androgynous bodies, with a Peter Pan-like quality. It may be dyspraxic, or at best have trouble negotiating the physical world and its limitations, shown as lateness, clumsiness, and muddle.

Psychological Air: needs space: physical, mental, and emotional. It cannot take the rumbustiousness of Fire, the dullness and heaviness of

---

[1]Modern Bible scholars debate a more nuanced interpretation of λoγoς. However, as many generations of school children will attest, they were taught it was the word of God that "made the world", emphasizing the literal translation as an order from God.

Earth, and the super-sensitivity of Water. It needs the silence and expansiveness of the upper air, to make sense of and systematise its thoughts. It needs freedom more than power. Air loves novelty, resists permanence, and is always in flux. Air relishes the cut and thrust of argument and can be cruel or insensitive.

Emotional Air: Air distrusts feelings and is more interested in thoughts, logic, and things that can be classified. Emotions are confusing to Air as they cannot be easily ordered or understood, so they disregard these or fail to understand cues and subtleties. This lack of understanding can bring coldness, cruelty, and lack of compassion.

Lack of Air: is often shown by a lack of reflection and objectivity, an inability to co-operate with others (Air is very collegiate). It may show in poor judgement, dismissal of the intellectual, reactive and emotional, superstitious or blinkered. Lack of Air shows as resistance to new ideas and difficulty in adjusting to change. It can also cause a weakened nervous system and psychological problems such as multiple personalities, or schizophrenia, in which there is an apparent splitting between mental faculties.

Excess Air: can show the superficial mind: the chatterer and gossip, the dilettante. They may lack connection with reality, their nervous system may be overwhelmed, they might have obsessive thoughts, or be subject to fanatical ideologies. They worry, over think, and may suffer from nervous exhaustion.

Spiritual Air: is expressed by deep thought, by meditation, by conquering the lower mind and embracing the concept of the higher mind of abstractions, of systems of belief, of the multiplicity and interconnectedness of spirit. Air expresses and contacts the spiritual through music, mathematics, and philosophy. The contemplation of divine systems gives the peace and order that Air craves. Air, along with Fire, is Apollonian; they actively and consciously form life, whereas Water and Earth, represented by Dionysus, are unconscious and instinctual forces. Paracelsus gives sylphs to Air (like Ariel in Shakespeare's *The Tempest*), which can only be controlled by constancy and commitment (i.e. Earth).

Social Air: The most social of all the elements, Air loves to chat and throw about ideas, explore theories, tell jokes, gossip. They will have a wide circle of friends of all kinds and love the noise and bustle of crowds. Fire and Air are rising and expanding, while Water and Earth are sinking and inert.

Sanguine temperament

The most socially acceptable of the four humours in Western culture, sanguine relates to youth, being both hot and moist. It is outgoing, warm-hearted from the Fire but also empathetic and people-focused, like Water. Sanguine is light, airy, optimistic, freedom-loving, larger than life, and has bigger plans and wider horizons than the other three humours. Sociable, energetic, humorous, affable, easy-going and some-times greedy, the sanguine person is the classic extravert who adores the crowd, the party, and loves to roam. Physically, sanguine people are great travellers, and also intellectually. Sanguine represents higher edu-cation, philosophy, astrology, spirituality rather than religion (which is melancholic with its rules and dogma, or phlegmatic in the sense of mysticism and union with the divine).

Physical characteristics

The damp quality plus the heat gives great expansion, so that often they are larger than life, tall, fleshy, with a tendency to put on weight. They have a good, ruddy complexion, lots of lustrous hair, red cheeks, a firm handshake, and warm, moist skin. Culpeper writes:

> A Man or Woman in whose Body heat and moisture abounds, is said to be Sanguine of Complexion, such are usually of a middle Stature, strong composed Bodies, Fleshy but not Fat, great Veins, smooth Skins, hot and moist in feeling, their Body is Hairy, if they be Men they have soon Beards, if they be Women it were rediculous to expect it; there is a redness intermingled with white in their Cheeks, their Hair is usually of a blackish brown, yet somtimes flaxed, their Appetite is good, their Digestion quick, their Urine yellowish and thick, the Excrements of their Bowels reddish and firm, their Pulse great and full, they dream usually of red things and merry conceits. (Culpeper, 1652, p. 52.)

Emotional characteristics

Like the element Air, sanguine types are warm but also distant; they like crowds and people but are less keen on intimacy or very emotional displays. They have moistness, so do understand feelings, but their fiery nature means they prefer action, shared with good company. They are the most content of the signs. Their optimism and geniality are hard to dent. Their airy nature soars above, regards from a distance, and is everywhere and nowhere and hard to pin down. Culpeper says:

> [T]hey are merry cheerful Creatures, bounteful, pitiful, merciful, courteous, bold, trusty, given much to the games of Venus, as though they had been an Apprentice seven yeers to the Trade, a little thing will make them weep, but so soon as 'tis over, no further grief sticks to their Hearts. (Culpeper, 1652, p. 53.)

In health

"Excess" is the word for sanguine; they generally are high-energy people, who can eat and drink mostly what they want. As Culpeper says: "They need not be very scrupulous in the quality of their Diet, provided they exceed not in quantity, because the Digestive Vertue is so strong" (Culpeper, 1652, p. 53). Sanguine warmth and moistness are excellent for the body and they tend to be robust and strong. Both physically and emotionally they are resilient and self-healing.

In sickness

The same excess can cause physical problems. However strong your constitution, eventually overdoing the eating and drinking and burning the candle at both ends will take its toll. The sanguine temperament shows especially in liver conditions, energy issues, respiratory problems, fleshy growths.

Regimen for sanguine

As the temperament with the strongest constitution, to stay healthy sanguine can eat pretty much anything and keep well with a minimum of exercise. A bit like phlegmatics, emotions play a strong part in keeping sanguine well. However, for sanguine it is feeling free and happy and interested in their world that keeps their emotions on an even keel. Sanguine likes novelty, fun, and stimulation for body, mind, and spirit. It is always a warning sign when a sanguine person isn't learning something new or breaking new ground in some way. Stagnation is their enemy, hope and enthusiasm their key to health. Alcohol and exercise can cause health problems:

> Excess in small Beer engendreth clammy and sweet Flegm in such Complexions, which by stopping the pores of the Body, engenders Quotidian Agues, the Chollick and Stone, and pains in the Back. Inordinate drinking of strong Beer, Ale, and Wine, breeds hot Rhewms Scabs and Itch, St. Anthonies fire, Quinsies, Pleuresies, Inflamations, Feavers, and red Pimples. Violent Exercise is to be avoided because it inflames the Blood, and breeds one-day Feavers. (Culpeper, 1652, p. 53.)

Culpeper on the signs of sanguine abounding

> The Veins are bigger (or at least they seem so) and fuller than ordinary; the skin is red, and as it were swollen; pricking pains in the sides and about the temples; shortness of breath; headach; the pulse great and full; urine high coloured and thick; dreams of blood &c. (Culpeper, 1653, p. 62.)

The Air signs ♊ ♎ ♒

Gemini ♊

Nature

Gemini is an Air sign, hot and moist, sanguine and mutable. Gemini is a sign of polarity, the two twins, so has a dual or two-faced nature. Geminis are great teachers and communicators, friendly, outgoing, intelligent, and quick. They can also be conmen, liars, and thieves, for what is truth anyway? They can see both sides of an argument or position, and can adopt either, hence their reputation for dishonesty, which may in fact be more like an attitude that there is not one truth but many. They have a magpie-like attraction to shiny bits of knowledge, which may make them informed, but not deep thinkers; communicators, but not philosophers. For this reason they make good journalists (anything to get the story), and politicians (very persuasive and adept at presenting "alternative facts"). Great entertainers, they can be all things to all people. Lilly adds: "active body, good piercing hazel eye, and wanton, and of perfect sight, of excellent understanding, and judicious in wordly affaires" (Lilly, 1647, p. 95).

Famous Geminis

Boris Johnson, Marilyn Monroe, Bob Dylan, and Alice Bailey.

Dignity and debility

Gemini is ruled by Mercury. Saturn is dignified in Gemini, Jupiter is in fall. Gemini is a sign of the spring. It is a barren sign and a humane or courteous sign.[2]

Physical

Gemini gives tall, slim bodies, a young, child-like demeanour, with small hands and feet, active and restless. Gemini rules the hands, arms and shoulders, and (with Jupiter) the respiration and the lungs. It rules the senses generally, but especially hearing and seeing. Gemini rules the brain and nervous system.

Emotional

Gemini is nervous, a chatterer and flighty. They may be disconnected from their feelings. Their mind working overtime can cause anxiety and insomnia. Lilly gives "distempered fancies" (Lilly, 1647, p. 94) to Gemini. They are great flirts, and are curious and friendly, but run a mile from deep emotional contact. They prefer to float above difficulties or simply move on if a situation becomes too "sticky". For this reason they have a reputation for being capricious, but deep and meaningful is not what they are about.

Mental

Overthinking, jumping from one thing to another, but sharp, quick, funny, open-minded, curious, always seeking the new information,

---

[2]Lilly says of the sign of Gemini, Virgo, or Aquarius ascending or Lord of the Ascendant: "we may judge the man to be of civil carriage, very affable and easie to be spoken with etc." (Lilly, 1647, p. 90).

new crazes, new stimulation. Twitter was made for Geminis: quick, verbal communication.

Illnesses

If a sickness is shown by Gemini, look to the emotions first as physical symptoms are often the way they process emotions. "When they fail to pace themselves properly they will be slowed down through accidents or falls that produce broken bones, strains or injuries mostly to the hands, arms or shoulders" (Watters, 2003, p. 35). Otherwise, Gemini shows coughs, other lung conditions, diseases of the nervous system, conditions affecting the hands and arms, trapped nerves, intermittent twitches, and tics. Sometimes muscular sclerosis or Parkinson's disease.

Treatment

Talking will be a help, any kind of talking cure. Their physical symptoms may chop and change due to the mutable nature of Gemini. Pacing themselves or finding a physical outlet for their mental energy is advisable.

Libra ♎

Nature

Libra is cardinal air, hot and moist, sanguine and masculine.

Famous Librans

Margaret Thatcher, Gandhi, Oscar Wilde, Edward Bach (of the Bach flower remedies), Louise Hay, and Deepak Chopra (see p. 244).

Dignity and debility

Libra is ruled by Venus. Saturn is exalted in Libra and Mercury is dignified. The Sun is in fall and Mars in detriment. It is a humane sign, and a sign of spring and childhood.

Physical

Ruled by Venus, Libra is one of the more beautiful signs of the zodiac. Even if they don't have classically attractive features, Librans have a grace and charm and allure which is hard to ignore or resist. Lilly says Libra has, "a round, lovely and beautiful visage" (Lilly, 1647, p. 97). Usually they have a slender body, with long limbs, a round face, big hair and an arresting gaze. Libra rules the kidneys and water balance in the body. They often have a pleasant, sweet voice.

Emotional

As an Air sign, Libra is a little cool and detached where feelings are concerned. Libra likes to talk about them rather than feel them too deeply; often they express their emotions through their creativity: music, art, poetry, and dance. Which is not to say they are not emotional; Libra likes harmony, but, in my experience, is the least harmonious of the signs, simply because their standards are so high and they hate to be disappointed. Annoy a Libran and you will unleash a torrent of emotion expressed verbally, which may well go on and on and on.

Mental

Despite being ruled by Venus, Saturn is exalted in Libra and this is expressed by their fine minds. They can forensically dissect any argument, see both sides and wear down an opponent by logic and sheer persistence. Lawyers, especially barristers, are shown by Libra, and also politicians: they excel in debate and can be ruthless opponents.

Illnesses

Libra shows kidney diseases, such as kidney stones, cystitis, urethritis. The back is an area of weakness and they often suffer from low back pain, lumbago, sciatica. Culpeper writes:

> Under Libra are diseases of the reines or kidnies which you please; for the significations of the word are the same; heat of the reines in women, which sometimes causeth death in travaile, many times abortion, always hard labour; the stone or gravel in the reins. (Culpeper, 1651a, p. 92.)

The sanguine humour rules the blood and Libra may show "corruption of the blood" (Lilly, 1647, p. 96) which occurs in recurrent infections.

Venus's love of sugar can cause problems with Libra's legendary lack of restraint; diabetes types one and two are shown by Libra.

Treatment

Loving luxury, Libra will respond well to aromatherapy, massage, and sweet-tasting remedies such as rose and orange blossom. They dislike exercise, so suggest dancing if weight needs to be shifted, or if back problems are caused by a sedentary lifestyle. They will like to talk about their ailments and to discuss and analyse your treatment plan.

Aquarius ♒

Nature

Aquarius is fixed air, sanguine, warm and moist, masculine, rational and humane. Traditionally ruled by Saturn, latterly Aquarius is co-ruled by Uranus. Mercury is in dignity while the Sun is in detriment.

Famous Aquarians

Germaine Greer, Oprah Winfrey, Bob Marley.

Dignity and debility

Aquarius is co-ruled by Saturn and Uranus. Saturn is exalted in Aquarius, Mercury is dignified and the Sun is in fall. It is a humane sign, ruling winter and old age.

Physical

Aquarius rules the legs, thighs, and ankles. As the sign of Uranus, there is often something unusual about the way an Aquarian looks or presents themselves which is part of the expression of their unconventional nature. Saturn, as ruler, gives a strong body; not attractive, but intense.

Emotional

The coolest of the Air signs, Aquarius can appear humble and modest, but it knows its value (Saturn) and uniqueness. Seen as eccentric,

Aquarius is not conventionally unconventional, but its own singular version of itself. Aquarius dislikes huge displays of affection, and noise and bustle, but prefers to stand back and observe rather than be in the mosh pit. It has a big heart, but generally for causes rather than individuals. Aquarians are fighters at the barricades of ideas and at the cutting edge of culture. They wish for justice for everyone, harmony and co-operation, world peace and brotherhood. Personal relationships may suffer as their focus is elsewhere, Aquarius will need to be friends with any romantic partner before they commit to a relationship.

Mental

The intellectual Aquarian is a seeker-out of philosophies that will improve the world, and they may even make their own up. Broad-minded, they can be critical, and dishonesty disgusts them. They have no time for time-wasters or laggards as they are on a mission and carry no passengers. They are often visionaries, before their time, waiting for the world to catch up with them. They can be blunt, their put-downs withering, but generally they are above pettiness and avoid discord and "difficult" people. Their fine minds incline them towards science and philosophy.

Illnesses

Any diseases of the legs and thighs and especially the ankles are shown by Aquarius. It also rules diseases of the veins, like varicosities, cramps, bruising. Due to their high standards and utopian outlook, Aquarius can be disappointed by real-world conditions; depression, pessimism and gloominess can be problematic. Culpeper says:

> Under Aquarius are all diseases incident to the Leggs and Ankles; all melancholy coagulated in the blood, cramps; and the truth is, thicknesse of blood most usually proceeds from this signe. Aske old Saturne and he will tell you the reason. By this the ingenuous have a plaine way to find out more; and by this Doctor Experience got materials to worke with. (Culpeper, 1651a, p. 94.)

Treatment

Although acupuncture pre-dates the discovery of Uranus by thousands of years, for me it seems to fit as a remedy for conditions shown by Aquarius because it involves the movement of energy in the body through subtle channels. Aquarians will accept the unusual if it fits into their mindset, so healing modalities such as radionics, reiki, and crystal therapy will appeal. Aquarians dislike touch, so they will not suit massage or other hands-on therapies. They will appreciate a logical analysis of their condition.

Temporary conditions

Heat

Causes

Summer, hot baths, poultices, burns, etc. Infections. Movement, exercise, hot food and drink. Emotions such as anger, wakefulness, insomnia, immoderate joy, overwork, worry.

Symptoms

Body feels hot.
Excess thirst.
Exhaustion.
Fever.
Burning and irritation in the stomach.
Burning urine.
Stabbing pain.
Bitter taste in the mouth.
Comfort in cold things.
Intolerance of hot food.

Itching skin, rashes.
Irritability.
Haemorrhage.
Dreams of heat and fire.
Insomnia.
Constipation.
Dry skin.
Dislike of the heat.

Cold

Causes

Excess rest and sleep.
Overeating dairy and sweet foods.
Cooling drinks and medicine, and cold food in winter.
Excessive heat, such as saunas, which disperse the inner heat and chill the body.
Fasting.
Build-up of humours that douse innate heat.
Chills.

Symptoms

Weak digestion, bloating.
No desire to drink.
Weak joints.
Catarrh and phlegm, sinus problems.
Dull, constant pains.
White discharges.
Lethargy, depression and fearfulness.
Aversion to cold food.
Diarrhoea.
Dislike of winter.

Moisture

Causes

Baths, especially after meals.

Moistening food and medicine.
Retention of matter usually excreted from the body.
Evacuation of dry humours.
Excess rest and sleep.
Things that cool the body, causing the humours to be retained.

Symptoms

A liking for abnormal cold.
Over-relaxation.
Excess saliva and secretion.
Diarrhoea and dyspepsia.
Excess sleep.
Water retention, swelling.
Dislike of winter and rain.

Dryness

Causes

External cold, which congeals humours and constricts the channels in the body and obstructs moistening nutrients.
Excessive heat, which disperses moisture.
Drying food, hot food, fasting.
Excess exercise.
Insomnia.
Emotional upset, anger.
Excess sex.

Symptoms

Dry skin.
Insomnia.
Wasting.
Intolerance of dry foods.
Desire for liquids and moist foods.
Dislike of autumn.
Skin absorbs readily.
Constipation and dry, hacking cough.

The seven natural things

SPIRIT			
THE FOUR ELEMENTS			
Fire	Earth	Air	Water
THE FOUR COMPLEXIONS (TEMPERAMENTS)			
Choleric	Melancholic	Sanguine	Phlegmatic
THE FOUR HUMOURS (FLUIDS)			
Choler	Melancholy	Blood	Phlegm
THE FOUR ORGANS			
Gallbladder Mars ♂	Spleen Saturn ♄	Liver Jupiter ♃	Lungs Moon ☽
THE FOUR OPERATIONS/ADMINISTERING VIRTUES			
Attractive hot & dry	Retentive cold & dry	Digestive warm & moist	Expulsive cold & moist
THE FOUR FACULTIES			
Vital	Animal	Natural	Procreative

1. SPIRIT—the organising principle.
2. THE FOUR ELEMENTS
    a. Fire and Water active: heat and cold.
    b. Air and Earth passive: moist and dry.
3. THE FOUR COMPLEXIONS (TEMPERAMENTS)
    a. Choleric: Mars ♂ and Sun ☉.
    b. Phlegmatic: Moon ☽ and Venus ♀.
    c. Melancholic: Mercury ☿ and Saturn ♄.
    d. Sanguine: Jupiter ♃.
4. THE FOUR HUMOURS (FLUIDS)
    a. Bile: choleric.
    b. Blood: sanguine.
    c. Phlegm: phlegmatic.
    d. Black bile: melancholy.
5. THE FOUR ORGANS
    a. Gallbladder: Mars ♂.
    b. Lungs: Moon ☽, Venus ♀.
    c. Spleen: Saturn ♄.
    d. Liver: Jupiter ♃.
6. THE FOUR OPERATIONS/ADMINISTERING VIRTUES
    a. Attractive—Choler—Mars ♂, Sun ☉—hot and dry.
    b. Digestive—Sanguine—Jupiter ♃—hot and moist.
    c. Retentive—Melancholic—Saturn ♄—cold and dry.
    d. Expulsive—Phlegmatic—Moon ☽, Venus ♀—cold and moist.
7. THE FOUR FACULTIES
    a. The Procreative Faculty—the reproductive organs—Venus ♀.
    b. The Natural Faculty—liver and veins—Jupiter ♃.
        i. blood—liver—Jupiter ♃.
        ii. phlegm—lungs—Venus ♀, Moon ☽.
        iii. choler—gallbladder—Mars ♂.
        iv. melancholy—spleen—Saturn ♄.
    c. The Vital Faculty—heart and arteries—Sun ☉.
    d. The Animal Faculty—nerves—Mercury ☿.
        i. Intellective
            1. Memory: Saturn ♄ cold and dry.
            2. Judgement: Jupiter ♃ warm and moist.
            3. Imagination: Mercury ☿ cold and dry.

ii. Sensitive
   1. Common sense: Mercury ☿.
   2. Sight: Sun ☉, Moon ☽, cold and moist.
   3. Taste: Jupiter ♃, hot and moist.
   4. Smell: Mars ♂, hot and dry.
   5. Hearing: Saturn ♄, cold and dry.
   6. Feeling: Venus ♀, all four qualities.

Herbs and the planets

The virtues of a Herb are its strengths and qualities; its inner potency, expressions of its Vital Spirit and of the way it is in the world. The way a herb is in the world will show the way it works in your body. We prefer this term to the more modern term "uses". Herbs do not have uses. They have themselves and their own purposes. (Private conversation with herbalist Christopher Headley.)

Saturn ♄

Rulerships

Saturn rules Capricorn and co-rules Aquarius with Uranus. He is exalted in Libra and in fall in Aries, and in detriment in Cancer and Leo. Saturn takes about twenty-nine years to travel around the zodiac. The Saturn return is often when reality bites, a time for marriage, divorce, life-changes, or when a person lets go of the life their parents wished for them and begins to build their own. These issues may also present as physical and emotional illness, so it is useful to look out for Saturn cycles.

Nature

Saturn is cold and dry, the greater malefic (Mars is the lesser malefic). Generally, in any horary or decumbiture chart, Saturn indicates negative influences. His friends are the Sun and Jupiter and Mercury, and his enemies are Mars and Venus.

Physically

Being cold and dry, generally Saturn shows thin, bony, hairy, often unprepossessing people. Their skin might be sallow, and their hair dark and stringy, what Lilly calls "a lumpish, unpleasant countenance". They often have a bent, crooked demeanour, "knees and feet indecent" (Lilly, 1647, p. 58). Saturn rules the bones, especially the knees and ankles, the right ear, the teeth, and the spleen.

Well dignified

Saturn gives great intelligence, and is often found in writers, academics, and scientists. They are silent, slow-moving, austere, courteous, conventional, measured, mature, and responsible. Saturn gives great strength and stamina.

Poorly dignified

A poorly dignified Saturn may show a person who is envious, paranoid, scheming, devious, calculating, jealous, mistrustful, ambitious, secretive, mean, stubborn, complaining, miserly, hard, cruel, misogynist, and selfish.

Illnesses

Saturn shows diseases of the bones such as arthritis and osteoarthritis. Saturn rules toothache, earache (the right ear; Mars rules the left ear), deafness, hard swellings (such as gall stones and kidney stones), consumption, wasting diseases, paralysis (with the Moon), gout, trembling, fainting, dizziness, fear, depression, psoriasis, and other disfiguring skin conditions. Lilly gives Saturn to: "all agues proceeding of cold, dry and melancholic distempers … vaine fears and fancies" (Lilly, 1647, p. 59). Culpeper writes:

> These diseases Saturne causeth by Sympathy; Tooth-ach, broken bones; the reason is because he rules the bones. Deafnesse he cavs-eth because he rules the eares. Melancholy and all diseases of the spleen by the same argument. Also, he afflicts all the parts of the body that are under the Moon by antipathy; and likewise he plays the same tricks with those that are under the Sun; you shall know what they are by and by. The great wisdom of a Physician is to know whether Saturne cause the disease by Sympathy or antipathy, and then take nothing, that as the cause is so is the cure, Sympa-thetical, or antipathetical; and withall do not forget, that sympa-thetical cures strengthen nature; antipathetical cures, in one degree or another weaken it. (Culpeper, 1651a, p. 85.)

Miscellaneous

Saturn rules Saturday, and the first and eighth hour after sunrise. It rules old age and autumn. Saturn rules religion rather than spirituality (which may come up in consultations). Saturn is happy in the first house, the eighth and the twelfth.

Herbs of Saturn

General characteristics of Saturn herbs.
Appearance: "ill-shaped, ill-smell, binding taste, lean, in filthy woody, solitary, dark places" (Culpeper, 1798, p. 20).
Element: Earth
Temperament: melancholic.
Qualities: cooling and drying.
Function: retention.
Organ: spleen.
Realm or virtue: memory.
Sense: hearing.
In this book: Bistort, Fumitory, Turkey Tail Mushroom, Witch Hazel.
In *A Woman's Book of Herbs* (Brooke, 2018): Comfrey, Horsetail, Shep-herd's Purse, Mullein.

In Culpeper: Hemlock, Mandrake, Mushrooms, Nightshade, Aconite, Henbane.

Bistort *(Polygonum bistorta)*

Saturn.
Cold dry 2/3.
Chakra: root.
Part used: leaves in summer, root in autumn.
Other names: snake weed.
Culpeper virtues: hardening, binding, thickens humours, cold and dry, absorbs moisture, reduces perspiration, cools the stomach.
Modern virtues: styptic, astringent.

History

Bis ("twice") *tort* ("twisted") relates to the appearance of the root. Steeped in water and roasted, Bistort is eaten in Nordic countries, ground into grain and baked into bread (Grieve, 1977, p. 105). The young leaves are made into a herb pudding in Cumberland and Westmoreland with nettles and dock leaves in early spring, when green vegetables are hard to find (Grieve, 1977, p. 107). Culpeper writes on how both the root and leaves powerfully resist poison and are used to expel the harmful humours of measles, chickenpox, and other infections, by inducing a great sweat (Culpeper, 1798, p. 87). He also recommends the decoction to stop any fluxes (discharges) in both men and women, that is, bleeding, phlegm and vomiting, etc. He writes that Bistort dissolves the congealed blood of wounds and bruises, reducing the pain this causes. He suggested taking the powdered root in wine to stop a threatened miscarriage. Likewise, the powder is helpful when spread on the gums of loose teeth to toughen up spongy gums. Finally, he recommends Bistort to dry up catarrh and phlegm in the head and treat tonsillitis and inflamed sore throats and vocal cords (Culpeper, 1798, p. 88).

Modern virtues:

Grieve gives a whole host of recipes using Bistort, which she describes as "one of the strongest astringent medicines" (Grieve, 1977, p. 106).
    Gargle for ulcerated tonsils (Grieve, 1977, p. 106):

Add 3.5ml of tincture of both Bistort root and 3.5ml of Bloodroot (*Sanguinaria*) (although I would use an equal amount of Shepherd's Purse instead), to 2 tbsp of warm water. Use as a gargle or spray.

For haemorrhoids (after Skelton, see Grieve, 1977, p. 107), use 15g of Bistort and 15g of Cranesbill. Boil and simmer for one hour, then make into an ointment with beeswax and other waxes, or mix into a gel. Apply locally. This will also be helpful to dry up herpes or boils on the face and body. (It may be too strong for genital herpes, though).

This final recipe is for infant diarrhoea (after Skelton, see Grieve, 1977, p. 107). 28g of Bistort root, 7g Cloves, 14g Marshmallow root, 7g Angelica powder, 7g Ginger powder. Crush the roots and cloves, boil in 850ml of water, and simmer down to 500ml. Pour onto the powder, mix and simmer for ten minutes. Cool, and add equal parts sugar or honey to make a syrup. Dose: 3–6 teaspoons daily in Raspberry Leaf tea.

Bistort is useful to cool and dry external or internal conditions which are caused by heat or moisture; so, diarrhoea, discharges, fevers with debilitating sweats. It may be helpful in menopause where there is flooding and sweating and weakness. It cools the brain in hot head-aches, insomnia, and panic attacks. Bistort is a great remedy for first aid kits, in powder form or, as a tincture, to stop bleeding, dry up pus, stop vomiting, etc.

Emotional

Bistort has the quality of emptiness; it is still, sinking, and dull. It gives a respite from mental chatter, fears, and unwanted thoughts. It is calming and cooling and centring to the emotions, grounding them in the earth. Use when rest and emptiness is needed, to empty the emotions in order to support the heart and mind for healing to begin. Use after trauma, upset, fright, and any condition where the emotions have become over-whelming and unbearable. Bistort gives a breathing space of silence.

Magical

Being a herb of Saturn, Bistort helps earthbound spirits to move on and banishes traumatic memories that need to be released. Mixed with Frankincense, Bistort is used in prosperity magic and fertility spells, especially where there have been miscarriages. Keep by the bed or under the pillow to bring a deep, dreamless, restful sleep.

Ritual

Bistort is a herb of the wise crone and of Samhain. Burn the root or add it to your incense mixture to gather in the spirits of the departed, and then send them on their way gently and with love. After miscarriage, burn the incense or sleep with it under your pillow to send the spirit of the dead child to the spirit world, and, if you wish, use to invoke the spirit of the next baby-to-be. The stillness of Bistort brings being and not doing into a ritual space. Use as preparation to concentrate and ground energies, to still the mind and heart, and empty the emotions and thoughts before powerful rituals or vision quests. Use afterwards to fully return to your physical form after astral travelling or any work with the World Tree or Kundalini. Bistort is very ancient and powerful.

Bistort is a constitutional remedy for melancholic temperament, along with Comfrey.

Fumitory *(Fumaria officinalis)*

Saturn.
Cold 2 dry 2.
Part used: herbs and seed.
Other names: Earth Smoke.
Chakra: root.
Culpeper virtues: cools head, liver, spleen and bowels, opening, purges melancholy, clears the skin.
Modern virtues: diuretic, blood purifier, hepatic, tonic, cholagogue.

History

Culpeper writes: "it clarifies the blood from saltish, cholerick and malignant humours. It is useful for leprosy, scabs and itch" (Culpeper, 1798, p. 183). The dried herb and seed cure melancholy. Gerard writes that it "opens and cleanses by urine, removes the stopping of the liver and spleen, purifyeth the blood as a decoction or syrup and dries all cholerike burnt and hurtful humors and is a most singular digester of salt and pituitous [phelgmy] humors" (Woodward, 1636, p. 1089). Dioscorides writes: "it quickens the sight and expels bilious urine" (Gunther, 1968, p. 659).

Modern virtues

Fumitory is used in biliary colic, jaundice, and migraine due to hepatic congestion. It has a long tradition of being used externally for hot, itchy skin conditions, such as urticaria, eczema, and rashes. Fumitory has been found useful for scabies; apply locally and use with Burdock and Cleavers. Taken often, Fumitory may have sedative or even a narcotic effect. It is used in cosmetics as a facial tonic due to its relaxant qualities. It gives a lovely yellow dye.

Emotional

Fumitory is a remedy for people whose roots have been torn or uprooted, through immigration or family trauma and splits. Fumitory balances the melancholic temperament when the person has become hard, judgmental, or bitter, where their dreams have been squashed, by others or by themselves. It is also useful for limited thinking among cynics and negative thinkers; for elders who have become too dry and hard, or who have lost connection with the earth and the natural world; and for gypsies, wanderers, and travellers whose feet do not touch earth.

Magical

Fumitory connects to ancestral wisdom and the ancestors; use it for any deep work dealing with family patterns or ancestral trauma (from war or flight or abuse). Use as a smudge or burn it in cleansing rituals. Similarly, Fumitory is useful to ground people after powerful magical experiences, mixed with Comfrey and Dandelion. The other side of pessimism is good planning; Fumitory helps in strategy meetings as a tea, or just on the table. It is used to consecrate ritual tools and to protect and purify a new home. It is an ingredient in money and prosperity magic.

Ritual

Fumitory is associated with Samhain; witches throw the herb into fires to invoke spirits of the underworld. I also use its planning qualities in Candlemas rituals, to organise the year, and at Samhain to assess how things are going. Its sober, practical, grounded, and cautious energies are helpful in any act of service. It is a constitutional remedy for melancholic and melancholic/phlegmatic temperaments.

Turkey Tail Mushroom *(Trametes versicolor)*

Warming.
Mushrooms are grouped under Saturn (and also, I would add, Pluto and Capricorn).
Chakra: crown and perhaps the root.
Traditionally used in Chinese medicine.
Modern virtues: adaptogen, anti-viral, pre-biotic. Immune-boosting. Digestive. Helpful during chemotherapy and in recovering quicker from radiation therapy, post viral syndromes, exhaustion, or any viral condition that has established itself deep in the body and is hard to shift.

Emotional

Turkey Tail is serious, ponderous, responsible but kindly. It acts on the heart for people reluctant to take on power or unaccustomed to having control. It has the indifference of universal love, and teaches lessons on sadness, solitude, and regret. This plant has great, deep, teachings, but will not give up its secrets easily. Ancient as it is, it has nothing to prove; you have to prove you are worthy to receive the teachings.

Magical

This ancient, prehistoric energy goes deep underground. It has a biting, snapping energy, and is sharp, focused, implacable, unconcerned, and directed, but also has a restlessness, almost machine-like in its movements as it transforms the rotten, as, indeed, it transforms old tree stumps. It is heavy, earthy, enclosed and protected. It has a hard shell with an inner softness. It will douse fire, so use in Earth rituals, building rituals, burying rituals.

Ritual

Turkey Tail is especially useful in passage of time rituals, memorials, days of remembrance. It has the wisdom of Solomon and helps with deliberations, difficult decisions, banishments, sacrifice of a member for the integrity of the group; correct actions, but taken with sadness.

Turkey Tail embodies the loneliness of leadership, where hard and sometimes unpopular decisions must be made. Drink as a tea or burn as incense. Use in retreats and on solitary vision quests for perseverance and stamina.

Witch Hazel *(Hamamelis virginiana)*

Saturn.
Cold and dry 3.
Part used: bark and leaves.
Chakra: ajna.
Modern virtues: astringent, sedative, tonic, anodyne.

History

This naturalised tree was originally from the eastern United States and Canada. It was a Native American remedy for wounds, tumours, and swellings. The name probably comes from its use as a dowsing rod (which was considered witchcraft).

Modern virtues

Witch Hazel is an excellent remedy for haemorrhage, swellings, and bruises, taken externally as an ointment or internally as a tea or tincture. Its strong astringent action makes it a first aid remedy for dysentery, diarrhoea, and heavy periods. It has pain-killing properties and so is helpful for the external treatment of haemorrhoids, varicose veins, red and itchy eyes, skin rashes, and inflammation. It is also good locally for insect bites to reduce swelling and itching: mix it with Chamomile or Lavender. Use the tea as a mouthwash or gargle for sore throats and bleeding gums, mixed with Myrrh and Thyme. Use externally, at the back of the ear, for glue ear in children, mixed with Calendula. The decoction is a helpful facial wash for acne and greasy skin; its astringent action will close up open pores (a facial steam can be helpful here). Use after childbirth on cotton pads or as a spray to soothe and tighten any bruised area, especially the perineum, mixed with Calendula for healing. It is helpful in nappy rash, which is hot and itchy, again as a diluted, strained tea, on cotton pads or sprayed. For bruising, sprains, and pulled muscles, mix with Daisy or Comfrey (see below).

Emotional

Witch Hazel has a sylph-like, sharp, clear, cutting, drying, cleansing energy, like a cool breeze. Relentless and implacable, it clears through old matter, slicing through stuck energy, cutting through misery. It allows you to separate from past wounds and trauma.

Magical

Use for vision questing, lucid dreaming, clairvoyance. It has the coolness of the upper air. Sleep with it under your pillow for dreaming and visions of the future. It is also useful as a tea or incense in planning meetings, for seeing things how they really are.

Ritual

Use in group meditations, where deep mind is plotting the future, in strategy meetings, or in meetings to deal with problems where expulsion or splits are called for. It is always better to divide a group rather than to self-destruct where agreement cannot be reached. In this way you can split harmoniously and grow separately.

Constitutional remedy for sanguine humour.

Jupiter ♃

Rulerships

Jupiter is a masculine planet, hot and moist, airy and sanguine. Known as the Greater Benefic, what Jupiter touches brings luck and good fortune. Lilly says: "he is the author of Temperance, Modesty, Sobriety and Justice" (Lilly, 1647, p. 62). He takes twelve years to pass through all the zodiac and the Jupiter return (when it conjuncts the natal Jupiter) is a time of expansion and growth. He rules the spring, childhood, the blood, the liver, the hips. Culpeper writes:

> Judgment is seated in the midst of the Brain, to shew that it ought to bear rule over all the other Faculties; it is the Judge of the little world, to approve of what is good, and reject what is bad; it is the seat of Reason, and the guide of Actions; so that all failings are committed through its infirmity, it not rightly judging between a

real and an apparent good. It is hot and moist in quality, and under the influence of Iupiter. (Culpeper, 1651b, n.p.)

Dignity and debility

Jupiter rules Sagittarius and Pisces. He is in detriment in Gemini and Virgo, and exalted in Cancer. He is in fall in Capricorn. Jupiter likes the second, ninth, and tenth houses.

Physically

An upright, straight, tall bearing, People with strong Jupiter carry themselves with authority and a sense of grandeur or power. A fleshy sign, with a characteristic oval face and abundant reddish hair. Large, soulful eyes, generally attractive and notable, rather than beautiful. They have a warmth and openness about them which is appealing. They are generally large. They may be tall or corpulent, or both.

Well dignified

They are generous, noble, honourable, fair-minded, honest, open-minded, inclusive, renowned for good deeds, kind to women and children, open-hearted, religious and charitable, prudent, virtuous and kind. Lilly writes: "aspiring in an honourable way at high matters, in all his actions a lover of fair dealings, desiring to benefit all men, doing glorious things … sweet and affable conversation, wonderfully indulgent to his wife and children … full of charity and godliness, liberall, hating all sordid actions, just, wise, prudent, thankful, virtuous" (Lilly, 1647, p. 62).

Poorly dignified

Wastrel, surrounded by sycophants, hypocritical, religious for show but neither good nor honest. ignorant, careless, mistreats people, gross, and dull, "abasing himself in all companies, crouching and stooping where no necessity is" (Lilly, 1647, p. 62).

Illnesses

Jupiter rules the liver and so all diseases of that organ, and diseases due to liver congestion, such as varicose veins, poor digestion, gas, and nausea. Also: pleurisy, fevers, lung diseases, palpitations, cramps, corrupted blood, and all diseases from excesses of alcohol, food, and work. Culpeper writes:

> Jupiter they say causeth … all infirmities of the Liver and Veins, inflammations of the Lungs, Plurifies and other Aposthumes about the Breast and Ribs, all diseases proceeding of putrefaction of blood and wind, quinsies, feavers, and other diseases; which Authors either for want of witt, or super-abundance of ignorance are pleased to attribute to him. (Culpeper, 1651a, p. 86.)

Culpeper disagrees that Jupiter shows corruption of the blood: "For Saturne corrupts the blood by melancholy, and Mars by choler" (Culpeper, 1651a, p. 87). But I disagree with him here, because I have seen Jupiter showing poisoned blood.

Jupiter also rules Taste, and:

> Resides in the Pallat which is placed at the root of the Tongue on purpose to discern what food is congruous for the Stomack, and what not; as the Meseraik Veins are placed to discern what nourishment is proper for the Liver to convert into Blood; in some very few men, and but a few, and in those few, but in a very few Meats these two Tasters agree not; and that is the reason some men cover Meats that make them sick, viz. The Taste craves them, and the Meseraik Veins reject them: In quality hot and moist. (Culpeper, 1651b, n.p.)

Plants

Jupiter rules Cloves, Dandelion, Meadowsweet, Sage, Borage, Mace, Nutmeg, Betony, Lungwort, Red Clover, Melissa, Hyssop, Limeflower, Agrimony.

Miscellaneous

Jupiter rules Thursday and the first hour after sunrise and the eighth. "All planets except Mars are friends to Jupiter" (Culpeper, 1798, p. 17). Jupiter shows astrology; a strong Jupiter in a decumbiture chart showing the physician or medicine indicates the treatment will be successful

(Jupiter as the Greater Benefic) but that it may be costly, as Jupiter likes luxury.

Herbs of Jupiter

> Jupiter is a benevolent planet, moderately hot and moist, answering to the liver and the faculties thereof, some say he rules the lungs and sides, veins blood and digestive faculty. (Culpeper, 1798, p. 17.)

Herbs of Jupiter nourish and enrich the blood and liver. The liver controls the condition of the blood, metabolism of the body, and the growth of tissue.

General characteristics.

Appearance: They have a good taste and smell; are often reddish or sky-coloured; may produce oil; and their leaves are plain.

Element: Air.

Qualities: warm and moist.

Temperament: Sanguine.

Function: digestion.

Organ: the liver.

Realm or virtue: judgement.

Sense: taste.

Herbs in this book: Agrimony, Milk Thistle, Borage, Betony.

Herbs in *A Woman's Book of Herbs* (Brooke, 2018): Dandelion, Hyssop, Limeflower, Meadowsweet, Melissa, Red Clover and Sage.

Herbs in Culpeper: Asparagus, Avens, Bay Tree, Wood Betony, Bilberries, Bugloss, Chervil, Sweet Cicely, Cinquefoil, Endive, Houseleek, Liverwort, Lungwort, Oak, Red Roses, Jack by the Hedge, Succory, Milk Thistle, Almonds, Walnuts, Vine Tree.

Betony *(Betonica officinalis [Stachys betonica])*

Hot 2 dry 2.

Part used: herb.

Planet: Jupiter in Aries.

Culpeper virtues: heats head, lungs, and kidneys. Warming pectoral. Dries the heart. Opening, warming diuretic, loosening tension. Opens liver and spleen.

Modern virtues: cephalic, nervine, tonic, astringent, aromatic, alterative, digestive.

History

Antonius Musa, physician to Roman Emperor Augustus, wrote a book on Betony and, among its virtues, claimed it was effective against epidemics and was also a protection against witchcraft (Culpeper, 1798, p. 81). Musa recommends it for digestive stagnation (probably a cold stomach), with sour belching and griping pains in the gut, as it opens obstructions of the liver and spleen. He also recommends it for continual pains in the head, palsy, convulsions, and falling sickness or epilepsy. Musa recommends one drachm (approximately 2g) of the powder in a little honey and taken in vinegar for those who are over-wearied by travel. Culpeper writes, "it is a very precious herb, without doubt, and very proper to be kept in every house, preserved in syrup, conserve, oil, ointment and plaster" (Culpeper, 1798, p. 82).

Modern virtues

Betony is an excellent remedy for headaches, migraines, and brain fog, or any injuries to the head. It works best as a curative remedy rather than a first aid medicine. However, I have found mixing it with Wild Lettuce and Lavender or Rosemary (Brooke, 2018, pp. 199, 38) is fairly effective for headache. Betony comes into its own for the long-term treatment of chronic migraine, menstrual headaches, and following trauma to the head; take it as a tea or tincture. Like all conditions of the nervous system, Oats will provide a base for healing the nervous system with a more targeted remedy such as Betony. Betony also works on the digestive system, which is helpful with migraine, for example, where there is nausea and vomiting. Betony may be helpful in dementia or mental confusion, and also in post-stroke rehabilitation, but of course this will require the assessment of a skilful, trained herbalist. It is also used in neuralgia, combined with St. John's Wort, again taken as a curative rather than a first-aid remedy.

Emotional

Working on the head, Betony is useful for anxiety states caused by over-thinking, for people who try to over-intellectualise their emotions or to put them into rational boxes, where, of course, they do not fit and will pop out as anxiety, headaches, gut pain, palpitations, and diarrhoea. It calms the solar plexus, and moves the energy from there and also down from the head to the heart, where trust and peace are found. Use where the person feels "out of their body" for some reason, or "in their heads", to bring them back to physicality and nature. Betony is grounding, slow, and implacable. Use where people are "in their heads" but not where there is depression or gloominess (it is too dulling), particularly when there is difficulty in focusing and applying oneself to the task in hand. It is useful where people repeat negative patterns because they do not listen to their hearts, but operate from rational analysis (which, actually, is often irrational) or gut feelings, often driven by fear and lack of trust.

Magical

Traditionally Betony was used to prevent visions and dreams and to protect from evil spirits. To this end it was planted in churchyards and worn as an amulet to "drive away devils and despair" (Grieve, 1977, p. 97). As such, Betony is a remedy for protection and banishing ill-wishing. It is also used for journeying and connecting to spirit, bypassing the rational, limiting mind, and opening up to the wonders of spirit's wide-open vistas. It is a herb of the head (Jupiter in Aries) and builds bridges between lower and upper mind, grounding spiritual experiences while relieving a mind that is gloomy and stuck in the limitations of the rational.

Ritual

Use in rituals for fire moons, and also before travelling to give the courage and the energy to accomplish all one wishes to. Use in Beltane and Midsummer rituals for visioning the future and putting faith (Jupiter) in the benevolence (Jupiter) of the universe. It can be drunk as a tea or burned as incense.

Milk Thistle *(Silybum marianum)*

Hot 2 dry 2.
Part used: the seeds.
Culpeper gives thistles in general to Mars (for their sharp prickles) and Milk Thistle to Jupiter.

Culpeper virtues: draws choler by sympathy, melancholy by antipathy, hepatic, opening, cleansing, resists poisons, heat in the head and heart. Modern virtues: galactagogue, hepatic, demulcent, blood cleanser.

History

Milk Thistle opens the liver and is one of four herbs Culper recommends as true hepatics which cleanse the liver without heating it.[1] Gerard claimed it was the best remedy for melancholy. Culpeper recommended boiling the young plants (after removing the prickles) for a blood cleanser (Grieve, 1977, p. 797).

Modern virtues

One of my favourite herbs, useful for so many physical conditions where the liver needs support and healing. Especially useful in gynaecological disease where a sluggish liver is slow in breaking down hormones: premenstrual tension, menopausal symptoms, and infertility. An excellent remedy for any liver condition, taken as a tea or decoction: hepatitis, post-viral symptoms, acute and chronic infections, varicose veins (from hepatic congestion), lack of appetite, poor digestion, and nausea. Note that the seeds need to be extracted in alcohol of at least sixty-five per cent proof to be effective, or else take ground to power in capsules.

Emotional

The liver is concerned with the "digestion" of lower emotions. In depression, always treat the liver; it can help to release trapped anger in there and allow the tears to flow freely, which flushes out the liver. Milk Thistle is good where emotions are blocked, and the person is stuck in their life; it helps them to move on to the next stage. It is not helpful where there is too much anger and there is a need to cool down and withdraw energy from the liver. Likewise, Milk Thistle is unhelpful where there is no sense of direction and the person is stuck in misery. Here, more tears are not helpful; another kind of closing down is needed.

---

[1]The others are Wormwood, White Horehound, and Agrimony (Tobyn, 1977, p. 206).

Magical

Milk Thistle has much of the wise warrior about it, the young hero. It is useful for young men when they hit puberty, to contact their inner strength and connect with healthy masculine archetypes. It builds up resilience and inner strength to withstand the brain-washing of toxic masculinity. It can be taken as a tincture but also ground up as a condiment and added to food. It has a nutty, bitter taste. Milk Thistle can be added to maji (see p. 79) for courage and strength and focus.

Ritual

Use in rituals before a vision quest or a trial of strength, especially on the fire moons, Aries and Sagittarius. Use in ecstatic dance, power raising, and weather work. It has the quality of wild, noisy, foot-stamping, high energy. Use it to dance through blocks and obstacles, to shed old, outworn patterns, and ways of being; or to bind a group together after a dispute, around a fire, shouting, chanting, and raising energy, speaking your truth with a talking stick, telling hard, uncomfortable, angry truths. Use it before a big adventure, to connect the energies of heaven and earth, like a lightning rod to ground spiritual energy. It has strong masculine energy, and great power. Use it with sacred drums to call up wild spirits, such as banshees or earth spirits. It connects to the pulse of the earth, and summons chthonic energies; use it in sacred Earth rituals. It has a very powerful energy, so use it wisely and compassionately.

Milk Thistle is a constitutional remedy for sanguine, together with Borage, Melissa and Agrimony.

Agrimony *(Agrimonia eupatoria)*

Jupiter in Cancer.
Hot 1 dry 1.
Part used: herb.
Culpeper virtue: cleansing, cutting without any manifest heat, binding, heats liver, heart, spleen, kidney and bladder. Glutanating (joining together) and alexipharmic (poison antidote).
Modern virtue: astringent, tonic, diuretic, hepatic.

History

Agrimony comes from *Argemone,* a Greek word for the class of remedies which were healing to the eyes (Grieve, 1977, p. 13). *Eupatoria* refers to Mithridates VI Eupator of Pontus (120-63 BCE), a king renowned for his ability to withstand poison, which he developed by taking small doses to build up his immunity (Radice, 1973, p.167). It was used by the Anglo Saxons for wounds and snake bites. In Chaucer it was mixed with Mugwort and vinegar for back problems and wounds (Grieve, 1977, p. 14). Culpeper writes: "it opens and cleanses the liver ... is beneficial to the bowels, healing all inward wounds" (Culpeper, 1798, p. 53). Sores can be healed by bathing them in a concoction of Agrimony. Agrimony cures all diseases of Jupiter and Cancer by sympathy, and strengthens those parts ruled by these planets. It treats diseases under Saturn, Mars and Mercury, by antipathy, if they occur in a part of the body ruled by Jupiter or under the signs Cancer, Sagittarius, or Pisces. So, it is good for gout and oedema, internally or externally as an oil (Culpeper, 1798, p. 53). Culpeper continues: "it is hot and dry in the first degree; binding, it amends the infirmities of the liver, helps such as piss blood, helps inward wounds, opens obstructions; outwardly applied it helps old sores, ulcers &c. Inwardly it helps the Jaundice and the spleen" (Culpeper, 1653, p. 25).

Modern virtues

Agrimony is an excellent, gentle, liver herb, which nevertheless has a strong, sustained action to cleanse, strengthen, and tonify the liver. Use for recovery from hepatitis or glandular fever as a tea, or for any infectious disease, to increase elimination and boost immunity. It is excellent for children's diseases, such as chicken pox and measles, and as a remedy to cleanse the blood in acne and other skin conditions. It has a slight heating action, which helps when debility has set in post-virally, experienced as coldness and lethargy. It is an excellent wound-healer and is also excellent for bites, stings or sores. Use a strong decoction, or the fresh herbs in a poultice.

Emotional

Agrimony gives strength in solitude; its dryness sucks out soggy emotions to bring a feeling of leanness and austerity. It is like a lighthouse burning among the smoke and ruins of disaster; it allows you to regroup and bring back your strength. After a lot of crying it dries up the tears. Agrimony helps to overcome inner blocks. It prevents escapism and brings the person back to the essentials, which may be painful, but this is the only way to regain power. It is helpful for the over-relaxed or self-indulgent, such as phlegmatics. Agrimony feels a bit Saturnine, but it works like Jupiter to focus on the future, on hopes and dreams and plans; its austerity helps the person proceed with making these a reality. Use in sleep pillows for fear and nightmares. Agrimony is one of the Bach flower remedies, indicated for people who hide their pain behind a facade of cheerfulness, often over-using drink or drugs to deal with the pain they feel. Frequently, other people have no idea of the suffering they experience. Agrimony creates a protective barrier while healing occurs, a traditional remedy for returning hexes, Agrimony can be used to send back negative energy.

Magical

Agrimony's self-contained power is useful for vision quests and solitary journeys, for long journeys of exploration, both inner and outer. Use during big changes in life, to concentrate down to the essentials and to focus your energy so that nothing is wasted.

Ritual

Use in rituals to banish and let go after separation and break-up. Release those things that remind you of the person or circumstance, maybe burning letters or symbolic drawings of what the relationship represented to you. Do this at a full moon, where the energies are culminating. Dancing and chanting are powerful ways to shed burdens, history, and pain. Mix with Mugwort for healing and protection rituals.

Agrimony is a constitutional remedy for sanguine, together with Borage, Melissa, and Milk Thistle.

Borage *(Borago officinalis)*

Jupiter in Leo.
Hot 1 moist 1.
Part used: the herb.

Other names: Starflower.
Culpeper virtues: Refreshes the vital spirit, expels melancholy, comforts the heart, heats and moistens the heart.
Modern virtues: diuretic, demulcent, emollient, adrenal trophorestorative, anti-inflammatory, sedative, expectorant, adaptogen.

History

It is claimed that Borage steeped in wine was the legendary drink nepenthe, which Helen, rescued from Troy, gave to her husband Menelaus to forget all his sorrows. Henslow suggests the name Borage comes from the Celtic *barrach* meaning man of courage (Grieve, 1977, p. 120). The Latin tag *ego borago, gaudia semper ago* ("I am Borage I always bring happiness") suggests it drives away sadness, dullness, and melancholy. Gerard writes: "a syrup of the flowers quieteth the phrenticke and lunaticke person … exhilarate and make the mind glad … it is used for the comfort of the heart, to drive away sorrow and increase joy in the minde" (Woodward, 1636, p. 797). Dioscorides recommends it for the chills of acute fevers, for abscesses with Mullein and "put into wine, is thought to cause mirth" (Gunther, 1968, p. 677). Borage is one of Culpeper's four cordial flowers, which help the heart troubled by melancholy.[2] Bacon claimed it "hath an excellent spirit to repress the fuliginous vapor of dusky mancholie" (Grieve, 1977, p. 120). Culpeper describes Borage as one of the great cordials and strengtheners of nature. He recommends it mixed with Fumitory to cool, cleanse, and temper the blood for itchy skin conditions. He suggests always using the fresh herb (or perhaps a diluted fresh herb tincture) for red and inflamed eyes (Culpeper, 1798, p. 90).

Modern virtues

Borage is an excellent herb for treating exhaustion after surgery, prolonged stress and trauma, and chemotherapy. It gently nourishes and strengthens the adrenals to build up stamina slowly and safely. Use after flu to build up resilience and strength. It is soothing due to its high mucilage content and is a useful cough remedy, a good treatment for bronchitis and sore throats, colds and hoarseness. It can be used as

---

[2]With Viper's Bugloss, Rose, and Violet (Tobyn, 1997, p. 204).

a soothing demulcent for cystitis and gastritis. Borage, when taken as a tea, is a traditional remedy to increase the quality and quantity of breast milk, with its strengthening and stamina-building properties being a helpful adjunct.

Emotional

Borage, as the ancients said, gives courage. In a modern context this translates as giving the strength to keep going. It builds mental as well as physical stamina, excellent for "burnout" with Oats to nourish a depleted nervous system, and Rose to feed the heart that is exhausted. It is useful during the pressure of exams and in any prolonged, stressful situation. It can be used for the emotional strain of the menopause, especially where there is great sadness about the passing of fertility, together with insomnia or depression. Being a herb of Jupiter, Borage brings joy, a feeling of hope and optimism. It gives a sense of wellbeing and stillness, like an active peacefulness. After trauma and loss, Borage helps to begin to see a plan for the future and gives the strength to carry out that plan. It has a poised, tensile strength. It is warm, centred, and powerful. It calms fears with a sense of certainty and bringing the person back into the moment. Borage can be a herb for the maji mix, (see p. 127) to give courage and stamina and hope for change.

Magical

Use after shock, trauma, or long, debilitating illness to find your centre again. Burn as incense during meditation to focus on re-building vitality and strength. Use as tea in groupwork, to build a group heart connection during times of testing and dissent. For fearful children, use as an amulet around the bed and in pillows for a calm sleep. It provides protection in the between-times, for sitting and thinking and taking a breath from activity. Borage is a herb to aid the development psychic powers. It is also protective; sprinkle the infusion around to ward off bad energy.

Ritual

Borage contains the secrets of the upper air. It has the quality of floating and gliding above the land, above your issues, and allows you to look down on your life and see it for what it is. Borage gives perspective. It is helpful in the middle years, to evaluate life, and for menopause rituals or times of transition, leaving or moving home. It brings a quality of great peace and a sense of the calm beauty of life. Float Borage flowers in the bath before rituals and to raise energy.

Borage is a constitutional remedy for sanguine, together with Agrimony, Melissa, and Milk Thistle.

Mars ♂

Rulerships

Mars rules Aries (day time) and Scorpio (night). He is exalted in Capricorn (twenty-eight degrees) and in fall in Cancer. Mars does not do well in the signs of Venus, Libra, and Taurus.

Nature

Masculine, nocturnal, hot and dry, choleric and fiery (Lilly, 1647, p. 66). Mars is known as the Lesser Infortune, the greater is Saturn. Mars is the author of "quarrels, strife and contention" (Lilly, 1647, p. 66).

Well dignified

A strong Mars makes the person courageous, indomitable and competitive. Lilly says Mars is: "In feats of Warre and Courage invincible, scorning any should exceed him, subject to no Reason, Bold, Confident, Immoveable, Contentious, challenging all Honour to themselves, Valiant, lovers of Warre and things pertaining … hazarding himself to all Perils" (Lilly, 1647, p. 66). They are free thinkers who dislike being told what to do. Excellent in any emergency, they will take command, execute decisions, and cut through any red tape to get the job done.

Poorly dignified

The other side of such dynamism and power is that they are "willing to obey no body or submit to any; a large reporter of his own Acts". Argumentative, selfish, and aggressive, a strong Mars is hard to be around. Their huge egos are insanely competitive, selfish, and boastful. When crossed, Mars (the god of war) can be violent, aggressive, and cruel.

Lilly continues: "he is a prattler without modesty or honesty, a lover of Slaughter and Quarrels, Murder, Thievery, a promoter of sedition, Frayes and Commotions … as wavering as the Wind a Traytor, of Turbulent spirit Perhured, Obscene, Rash, Inhumane, neither fearing God nor caring for man, Unthankful, Treacherous, Oppressors, Cheaters, Furious, Violent" (Lilly, 1647, p. 66).[3]

Physically

Mars shows, strong, muscular bodies with a compact, athletic form. They often have a reddish or sandy-coloured hair and complexion, with a round, ruddy face and sharp, penetrating eyes with a bold stare. They are usually hot to touch and wear light clothing even in the coldest weather. They find it hard to sit still and are restless and irritable. They are "active and fearless" (Lilly, 1647, p. 67).

Illnesses

Mars rules the gallbladder, the left ear, migraine, any burning fevers, shingles, blisters, burns, rashes and pustules, and any disease of heat. Mars shows jaundice and diseases of the male reproductive system as well as conditions caused by wounds, accidents, "and other such diseases as arise by abundance of too much Choler, Anger or Passion" (Lilly, 1647, p. 67).

Herbs

Herbs ruled by Mars tend to be sharp, cutting, stinging, strong-flavoured and bitter. They grow in dry places and are "corrosive and penetrating the Flesh and Bones with a most subtill heat" (Lilly, 1647, p. 67). These include: Garlic, Onion, Chilli, Nettle, Thistles, Brambles, Ginger, Pepper, Leeks and Mustard.

Miscellaneous

Mars rules summer, Tuesday, and the first and eighth hour after sunrise. It rules youth and the third month of pregnancy (perhaps when

---

[3]Donald Trump has Mars conjunct his Leo Ascendant.

fighting for life begins?). Mars delights in the third, sixth, and tenth houses, has no friends other than Venus, and so is an enemy to all the other planets. "Mars is a friend to Venus and an enemy to all the rest" (Culpeper, 1798, p. 18).

General characteristics

Appearance: plants that are rough and prickly, reddish, have a burning taste, and grow in dry places.
Element: fire.
Temperament: choleric.
Quality: heating and drying.
Function: attraction.
Organ: gallbladder.
Realm or virtue: none.
Sense: smell.
Mars heats and dries all it comes in contact with. It resists poisons, dries up body fluids, and stimulates the body.
Herbs in this book: Basil, Nettle Seed, Garlic, Holy Thistle.
Herbs in *A Woman's Book of Herbs* (Brooke, 2018): Bearberry, Ginger, Hawthorn, Hops, Nettle, Vitex, Wormwood.
Herbs in Culpeper: Briony, Brambles, Broom, Toad Flax, Mustard, Horseradish, Rhubarb, Tobacco, Onions.

Basil *(Ocymum basilium)*

Mars in Scorpio.
Hot 3 and dry 3.
Chakra: solar plexus.
Part used: fresh leaves.
Culpeper virtues: resists poison, heating.
Modern virtues: expectorant, diaphoretic, drying, nervine, cephalic, anti-inflammatory, anti-oxidant, anti-bacterial, anti-fungal.

History

The name *basilium* possibly comes from the Greek βασιλευς or king. Parkinson suggests this may be because of the agreeable smell or because it was used as an unguent or remedy in the royal courts. Basil was associated with scorpions; Parkinson wrote that if the leaves were bruised scorpions would breed from them (Grieve, 1977, p. 87). In Culpeper's day, Basil was seen as a powerful herb that was rarely used internally except to help the deficiency of Venus and destroy her also (Culpeper, 1798, p. 75). He recommends Basil to expel the afterbirth and to bring on labour. It is also useful to draw out the poison of insect bites and stings. It is a sacred plant of Krishna and Vishnu in the Hindu tradition, and is kept in every house to purify the air.

Modern virtues

Basil is a powerful anti-inflammatory remedy. The oil is high in antioxidants, and so it is used in any chronic inflammatory condition and to boost immunity. The fresh leaves have anti-bacterial qualities and can be used locally for infected wounds. Heating and drying, Basil expels phlegm from the lungs and can be helpful in cold, mucous coughs, and catarrh; its anti-bacterial qualities make it helpful as a chest rub in bronchitis with Eucalyptus or Pine essential oils, or use in a steamer or oil diffuser in the sick room.[4] Basil is also a remedy for infected gums and toothache, applied locally. The oil is also used as a muscle relaxant, mixed with Rosemary or Lavender oil, or a couple of drops in a hot bath after strenuous exercise will untangle knotted muscles. Basil is anti-fungal and so is a useful remedy for athlete's foot and other persistent fungal infections, applied locally. Basil has been used in Ayurvedic medicine to heal ear infections, by rubbing the oil mixed with Frankincense behind the ears and on the bottom of the feet. Basil is also preventative and curative for insect bites; the essential oil applied locally on the bite will stop the itching and inflammation.

Emotional

Basil is an uplifting herb and so can be helpful in anxiety and low mood. It increases stamina and resilience by supporting the adrenal glands. Use a couple of drops on pulse points for exhaustion and tension headache. It can help remove unwanted thoughts and an over-active mind. It is

---

[4]Essential oils should never be taken internally unless under the guidance of an experienced aromatherapist. Always dilute in a carrier oil, such as Almond or Cocoa.

also a remedy for cold, dull, headaches brought on by crying or depression. Heating and drying, Basil can temper excess watery emotions to move away from victimhood and passivity. It calms the emotions where there are arguments and discord, allowing for calm discussion and conflict resolution. Basil helps to move energy from the solar plexus to the heart chakra, from reaction and defensiveness to love. It softens spitefulness and irritation and intolerance to create a healing fire, not a hurting fire.

Magical

Use to keep away toxic people who wish to harm because of their own pain. Hang on bedsides to remove night terrors and protection from wandering spirits. Basil makes a useful flower remedy (see p. 113) to build up the warrior spirit and to protect from strong influences. In India, Basil is said to balance the chakras and enhance physical and mental endurance. It is used in peace spells. In Vudu a strong tea is made of the Basil plant, which is sprinkled in the entrance of a home or business to draw money luck and repel conflict. Use for protection while travelling and to aid astral travelling and journeying.

Ritual

This is a strong, protective, banishing, and purifying herb. It could be used for psychic attack or, better, protection from the attacks of others. It gives great inner strength and potentises prophetic and psychic abilities. Use in Samhain rituals, to contact wild Hecate or before vision questing or dangerous enterprises, where Basil offers deep insight and strong protection from harm. Basil can be used in banishing rituals and also for hexing rapists and abusers.

Garlic (Allium sativum)

Mars.
Hot 4 dry 4.
Chakra: ajna.
Part used: the bulb.
Culpeper virtues: resists poison, heating, drawing, digestive, binding, opening, carminative.

Modern virtues: anti-microbial, anti-septic, expectorant, stimulant, dia-phoretic, anthelmintic, cardiac.

History

Garlic was put on stones at crossroads as a supper for Hecate (Grieve, 1977, p. 342). Culpeper writes that garlic expels tough phlegm, purges the head and helps lethargy, preventative against foul sores and ulcers, it mitigates against the effects of poisoning by bad water, chemicals, or poisons such as Henbane, Wolf's Bane, Hemlock, and other poisons. It is extremely good in all cold diseases, for dizziness, convulsions, and also is helpful for jaundice. He warns: "in choleric cases it adds fuel to the fire" (Culpeper, 1798, p. 187), in melancholy it extenuates that con-dition and can give strange visions and fancies. It also opens the lungs and kills worms in the belly.

Dioscorides writes: "it has a sharp, warming, bitter quality. It clears the arteries, either eaten raw or boiled, and lessens old coughs. A decoction in a hip-bath brings down menstrual flow and after birth" (Gunther, 1968, p. 307).

Gerard adds: "being eaten it heateth the body extremely, attenueth and maketh thin grosse humors, cutteth those that are thick and clammy, digesteth and consumeth them, also it opens obstructions and is an enemie to all cold poisons … but those of a hot complexion should abstain from it" (Woodward, 1636, p. 177).

Modern virtues

Garlic is widely used to keep blood pressure low and to reduce the like-lihood and of heart attacks caused by high blood lipids It is best taken raw, two to three times per week, or in capsule form. Some research has shown Garlic is helpful in certain types of cancers, including pros-tate, brain, and lung cancer. Garlic has had a positive effect on alcohol-induced liver disease. Garlic is a powerful anti-microbial, anti-septic remedy. I use it raw in bronchitis, influenza, coughs and colds to heat up the body to fight the infection and dry up the mucus secretions. It is especially good as an expectorant when the phlegm is tough and causes paroxysmal coughing. Garlic is hard on the stomach; when taking it raw, be sure to eat beforehand to line the stomach as it may cause cramping or vomiting. Use raw or in a syrup as a post-viral remedy to build energy back up and fight lethargy, low mood, and tiredness (which are cold conditions). Garlic is an excellent first aid remedy for infected wounds and bites; mash a peeled clove in a little honey and put on the wound to draw out the poisons.

Garlic syrup: Peel and mash good-quality, juicy garlic cloves to almost fill a glass jar. Add a handful of Fennel or Aniseed and other cough remedies if required. (These will help with any cramping that the garlic might cause.) Pour over honey or syrup (made 1:1 water to sugar) to cover the Garlic, filled nearly to the top of the jar. Allow to sit in a warmish place for a week or so. Take one tablespoon as required. (If needed quickly, mash one garlic clove with one dessert-spoonful of honey and swallow down with copious water.) Repeat hourly until the cough has eased and the wheezing has subsided. For post-viral conditions, use the same method and take four or five times a day until strength returns.

As a prophylactic take the equivalent of a fresh Garlic clove two to three times a week. Cooked garlic has fewer of the medicinal qualities. Garlic may also be a useful herb to use in a sitz bath or yoni steamer (see p. 120) where there is infection such a trichomoniasis, thrush, or pelvic inflammatory disease.

Emotional

The fiery nature of garlic provides courage, protection, energy, and will-power. It dries up the lethargy and indecision of phlegmatics and the negativity of melancholics. Take a dessert spoonful of the syrup daily until your energy and willpower returns. If you are being bullied carry some with you as a protective talisman. Garlic keeps the will strong.

Magical

A herb used to invoke Hecate, garlic absorbs and returns negative magic, envy, ill-wishing and harm. Use it for protection: hang a bulb inside the front door, or by windows, or in your car, tied with red thread. Put it in backpacks, suitcases, and cars when travelling to protect yourself and your belongings. Change the bulb every month and dispose of it in running water. Use it to mark out and protect sacred space if you feel under attack. Garlic invokes martial magic, blood magic. It is fierce and ruthless.

Ritual

Use in ritual on fire moons, especially Aries. Anoint the ajna chakra with the infused oil in rituals which involve directing the will (see Brooke, 2018, p. 144). Garlic increases focus, intention, clarity. Use before battles with the law, marches, resistance, sit-ins, to be brave and clear. However, it is best tempered with heart remedies such as Rose and Melissa, because it is important to keep the heart engaged to do the right thing in the right way.

Holy Thistle *(Carduus benedictus)*

Mars in Aries.
Choleric.
Hot 2 dry 2.
Chakra: solar plexus.
Culpeper virtues: heats head and heart, opening, cleansing, resists poison, strengthens attractive faculty.
Modern virtues: cholagogue, digestive, anti-microbial, anti-inflammatory, galactagogue.

History

The name comes from a legend that the thistle prevented the troops of Charlemagne from falling ill with plague. It was believed that a message from God showed them the remedy. Turner (1568) writes: "it is good for any ache in the body and strengthens the members … it helpeth the memory and amendeth thick hearing" (Grieve, 1977, p. 796).

Culpeper said: "it is a herb of Mars and helps the swimmings and giddiness in the head, because Aries is in the house of Mars. It is an excellent remedy against yellow jaundice and other infirmities of the gall, because Mars governs choler" (Culpeper, 1798, p. 111). It strengthens the attractive quality because this is ruled by Mars. It helps sores, boils, itches and bites because Mars rules them, and it does this by sympathy. By antipathy it cures venereal disease, it strengthens the memory, and improves hearing by antipathy to Saturn who has his fall in Aries. It cures disease of melancholy and adjusts Choler by sympathy to Saturn as Mars is exalted in Capricorn. It is excellent for headache and migraine, taken as a powder. It comforts the brain, sharpens the wit, and strengthens the memory. Good for stomach upsets, it stimulates the appetite. The powder "ripens and digests cold phlegm, purges and brings [it] up" (Culpeper, 1798, p. 112). The herb provokes great sweats and "expels all poisons ... and other corruption or infection which may hurt and annoy the heart" (Culpeper, 1798, p. 112). He recommends it as a cure for food or water poisoning, as it creates a "mighty sweat which cleanses the body" (Culpeper, 1798, p. 112). He also claims it helps trembling and paralysed limbs.

Gerard writes, "*it makes thin grosse and tough flegme ... it helps concoction in the stomacke and is right beneficial to the heart*" (Woodward, 1636, p. 1001).

Modern virtues

Holy Thistle is a powerful bitter and is used wherever the liver needs support; poor appetite, recovery from illness, hormonal conditions, post-viral weakness, menopausal symptoms, systemic infections, as well as conditions localised to the liver such a hepatitis, nausea, and jaundice. It is a powerful anti-microbial and anti-inflammatory herb. Holy Thistle has been used to increase breast milk, however it is best avoided in pregnancy.

Emotional

Use it to dry up dampness, to get things moving, to speed things up, and for post-viral blues, not real depression because it is too sharp and stimulating, very ungrounded and speedy, but helpful for sadness and despondency, loss of hope, emotional lethargy. It brings courage and energy to the heart, gives stamina and the ability to get going again after setbacks. It renews vitality and strengthens the spirit. It is loud and confident, with a touch of bullying, bulldozing energy, like a rhino in full charge, it gets things done. Use sparingly.

Magical

Holy Thistle is good to find your warrior spirit; burn it as an incense or use in the bath. Use for feats of strength such as vision questing, protesting, at camps and on pilgrimages, or in any situation that requires stamina and staying power. It is useful to bring courage and stamina for people having chemotherapy or any other debilitating medical pro-cedure. Use it sparingly and rarely. This is a high energy plant which is hard to control. The strong Mars energy may tip over into aggression and violence, if it is not used where there is physical exertion to drain the high energy generated. Helpful for melancholics who have become stuck but are grounded and strong enough to withstand the release of energy Holy Thistle brings. Overuse can cause exhaustion.

Ritual

It is sacred to Pan and brings psychic protection. Burn it as an incense before a new project to bring luck and help and the energy to see it through. It helps to clear your path and to keep your focus razor-sharp. Use in clairvoyance to obtain a clear vision of the future or insights into problems and difficulties. Its ability to cut through muddle is helpful to resolve difficult problems and situations, and for planning and seeing the path ahead clearly. Use it to energise a group that has lost focus and purpose. It is great before group dances and chants to raise energy, channel aggression, and break through an impasse, and also for rituals to honour the goddess of fire and warriors.

Nettle Seed *(Urtica urens, Urtica dioica)*

Choleric.
Hot 3 dry 3.
Mars.
Culpeper virtues: heats lungs, kidneys, womb. Opening, diuretic, astringent, antilithic.
Modern virtues: adaptogen, heating, drying, stimulating, hepatic.

Historical

Culpeper writes, "nettles consume phlegmatic superfluities in the body, which the coldness and moistness of winter hath left behind. Nettle seed provokes urine and expels kidney and bladder stone, kills worms in children and expels wind, some think they are only "provocative to venery" Nettle is a remedy against venomous creatures … poisonous qualities, hemlock, henbane, nightshade and other herbs that stupefy and dull the senses and lethargy" (Culpeper, 1798, p. 578). Maud Grieve writes the seeds are an antidote to Hemlock, Henbane, and Nightshade poisoning—being hot and stimulating they counter the cold life-sapping qualities of these poisons. The seeds in a wine tincture were used for ague or malaria or any fever which involves fever and shivering. The powdered seeds were used for goitre, and it was a traditional remedy for overweight and sluggish metabolism (which may be caused by hypothyroidism).

Modern uses

Nettle Seeds are adaptogens—that is, a remedy which supports the adrenals and helps to mitigate the effects of stress on the body. They burn off phlegm and increase energy in a sustainable way (rather than just stimulating and then exhausting the body like caffeine for example). However, I find their action to be strong; I am a sanguine type, and they are ideal for phlegmatics or melancholics, or temporary phlegmatic or melancholic conditions, to bring much needed fire into the body. Use in conditions of long-term stress and exhaustion, chronic fatigue, after viral illnesses, or whenever the adrenals need support. With choleric or sanguine people, Nettle Seed's fiery nature may be too intense, and they can cause insomnia, palpitations, and general over-stimulation. Nettle Seeds are also an excellent remedy for chronic kidney conditions, because they work as a trophorestorative. They are kidney-food for all kinds of kidney conditions, for both people and animals. Locally, Nettle Seed mixed with Rosemary can be helpful to relieve pain due to cold, especially osteoarthritic pain, and it helps sprains and pulled muscles, bringing heat and blood to the area. However, they are hot, so please do a small patch test before applying, to check your skin doesn't react adversely to the heat. Avoid in conditions caused by heat, such as rashes and boils, as these will be exacerbated.

Nettle seed energy balls

1 part nut butter or tahini.
½ part honey or agave (or more, if not sweet enough).
2–3 handfuls of dried Nettle Seeds.
Good quality cocoa or cacao, to taste.
Desiccated coconut to bind, or oats (anything drying).
Chopped nuts—any kinds.
Chopped fruits.

Maca powder (another adaptogen with similar contraindications to Nettle Seed—see above).

Mix nut butter and honey in a bowl. Pass the Nettle Seeds through a medium sieve twice and add to the mix. Add the cocoa or cacao to taste (cacao is fairly bitter; you will need more sweetener probably). Then add the other ingredients. The aim is to make golf-ball sized balls, which are not too sticky but hold together. Roll the balls in cocoa powder, coconut, or sesame seeds, and chill to firm up. Use for snacks, hikes, period days, exams, any time you need a pick-me-up.

Emotional

The seeds have the same effect as the herb but stronger. They can help with burnout and general debility and weakness, sadness, and loss of focus, giving an energy boost which also has the effect of boosting mood and bringing confidence and clarity. There is no evidence that they can become habit forming, except in the way anything can become a habit. Their action on the adrenals will boost mood but long-term use should be mediated with lifestyle changes to get to the root of the issue.

Magical

They are concerned with bravery and focus, and so the seeds could be used in a maji mix (see p. 127), or for vision questing, or other trials of stamina and discipline and focus; all good Martian qualities.

Ritual

Nettle helps to dispel darkness and fear. It strengthens the will and boosts reactivity and supports the handling of shocks or the unexpected. Use in banishing rituals to drive negative energies from homes, cars, or businesses. Useful in ritual before political action or trials of courage.

The Sun ☉

Rulerships

The Sun rules the sign of Leo, the sign of midsummer, and has its detriment in the opposite sign of Aquarius. It is well-placed in the other Fire signs, Aries and Sagittarius. The Sun is badly placed in the Water signs, especially Pisces, and Scorpio.

Nature

The Sun is the seat of the vital spirit. Culpeper writes: "[the Sun] produceth the vital spirits ... by which the whole universe is cherished"
(Culpeper, 1798, p. 16).

Physically

The Sun rules the heart and the circulation, especially the arteries.
It also rules the right eye in men and the left eye in women. The condition of the Sun tells us a lot about the patient. The Sun is weak either
by astrological sign or the house in which it is placed. The Sun aspected
by malefic planets, such as Mars and Saturn, can show the person has a
low vitality, that their natural energy (vital force) is low or depleted for
some reason.

Well dignified

The Sun is hot and dry, but less so than Mars. It is a masculine planet,
and if well-dignified it is considered to be a fortune (Lilly, 1647, p. 70).
Lilly says of the Sun that he is faithful, and:

> [H]as an itching desire to rule and sway where he comes, prudent,
> of incomparable judgement, of great majesty and stateliness, indus-
> trious to acquire honour ... usually speaks with gravity ... with
> great confidence and command ... and not withstanding his great
> heart, yet he is affable, tractable and very humane to all people ...
> one loving sumptuousness and magnificence and whatsoever is
> honourable. (Lilly, 1647, p. 70)

Poorly dignified

Lilly writes that a poorly dignified Sun shows a man who is: "Arrogant and proud, disdaining all men", has poor judgement and foresight, and is, "restless, troublesome, domineering,' he is a spendthrift
and foolish, wastes his patrimony, hangs on other men's charity,
thinks all men are bound to him, because a Gentleman born" (Lilly,
1647, p. 70).

Physically

Generally, a well-placed Sun shows a strong body, sometimes lean or running to fat. They often have blond or golden highlights in their hair, with a flushed face, a large, round forehead and prominent eyes, which are often piercing or in some way fascinating. They enjoy a strong constitution and a lot of stamina. They have charisma and a kind of animal magnetism that is attractive. They are often found at the centre of a crowd.

Illnesses

The Sun shows diseases of the heart and circulation including palpitations, fevers, angina, heart attacks, and sudden collapse. The Sun shows mania and sometimes bi-polar conditions. A poorly dignified Sun can be expressed as depression, low spirits, exhaustion, post-viral conditions, dizziness, fainting and general weakness and apathy. It may also give a weak spine and back problems as well as diseases of the eyes (the right eye in men, and the left eye in women). Culpeper gives diseases of the Sun as:

> Pimples and Burles in the face, afflictions of the heart; Heartburning, Tremblings, Faintings, Timpanies, sore Eyes, and diseases of the mouth; Cramps, all diseases of the Heart and their ascendents the Arteries, Stinking-breath, Catharr's, rotten Feavers. (Culpeper, 1651a, p. 81)

Herbs and plants

Solar plants are often yellow or reddish and have a pleasant smell and taste. They are usually plants that love light and direct sunlight. Lilly says: "Their principall Vertue is to strengthen the Heart, and comfort the Vitals, to clear the Eye-sight, resist Poyson and dissolve any Witchery or Malignant Planetary Influences" (Lilly, 1647, p. 71).

For example: Chamomile, Juniper, Centaury, Saffron, Laurel, Grapes, St John's Wort, Amber, Musk, Marigold, Rosemary, Cinnamon, Celandine, Eyebright, Peony, Barley, Cinquefoil, Myrrh, Frankincense, Orange, Lemon, Cedar.

Miscellaneous

The Sun rules youth, when the vital spirit is strongest. He rules the summer, Sunday, and the first hour of the day and the eighth hour. The Sun is friends with all planets except Saturn, who is his enemy. The Sun rules the fourth, ninth, and eleventh houses.

Culpeper writes that the Sun "produces the vital spirits ... by which the whole universe is cherished" (Culpeper, 1798, p. 20).

General characteristics

Appearance: plants of the Sun generally have a yellow flower, a good smell and taste, and like to grow in bright sunlight.
Element: fire.
Qualities: moderately hot and dry.
Temperament: choleric.
Function: attraction.
Organ: the heart.
Realm or virtue: the imagination, vital virtue.
Sense: sight with the Moon.
Herbs in this book: Angelica, St. John's Wort, Eyebright, Celandine.
In *A Woman's Book of Herbs* (Brooke, 2018): Centaury, Chamomile, Juniper, Marigold and Rosemary.
In Culpeper: Lovage, Peony, Pimpernel, Saffron, Walnut.
General qualities of Solar herbs: Support and nourish the vital spirit, the essential energy of the body.

Angelica *(Angelica archangel)*

Sun in Leo.
Hot and dry in third degree.
Chakra: the heart.
Parts used: roots, leaves, and seeds.
Culpeper virtues: diseases from cold in the lungs and the kidneys and bladder, warming, anti-inflammatory. Heats heart, joints, and womb. Alexipharmic.
Modern virtues: carminative, stimulant, diaphoretic, expectorant, tonic.

History

Angelica comes from the Greek Αρχαγγελος ("chief angel") and refers to the myth that the Archangel Michael showed humanity how to use the plant. Gerard writes, "Angelica is an enemy to poysins" (Woodward, 1636, p. 1001). Culpeper writes that Angelica: "Is hot and dry in the third degree, openeth, digesteth maketh thin, strengthens the heart, helps fluxes, and loathsomness of meat, it is an enemy to poyson and pestilence, provokes the terms in women, and brings away the afterbirth" (Culpeper, 1649, p. 25). Angelica is good against poison.[5] Poisons are generally cold in nature, such as Henbane and Hemlock, which kill by shutting down the vital spirit of the body. Culpeper recommended Angelica root to treat pestilence and to stop pleurisy, before the heat of inflammation enters the body. He suggested its use in diseases of the lungs and kidneys and bladder caused by cold. Angelica helps against gnawing pains from cold, such as dull headaches, dragging period pains, thick coughs. Angelica resists diseases of Saturn and poison by "defending and comforting the heart, the blood and spirits" (Culpeper, 1798, p. 60). A tincture in wine "eases the pains and torments of cold and wind … it opens the stopping of the Spleen and the Liver, eases inward wind and swelling" (Culpeper, 1798, p. 60). Culpeper recommends it for poor eyesight, bathing the eyes with the juice or distilled water; and for toothache, by packing the tooth with the root or juice of the herb. The juice and distilled water scour and cleanse old wounds. The water was used for gout and sciatica. It melts away tough humours which have been bound together (we might understand this as muscles and ligaments stiffened and tense). Culpeper suggests:

> [L]et it be gathered when the sun is in Leo and the Moon is applying in good aspect in the hour of the Sun or the hour of Jupiter. Observe the like in gathering the herbs of other plants and you may happen to do wonders. (Culpeper, 1798, p. 58)

Modern virtues

Angelica is excellent for fevers and cold and chills. Take the tea or tincture to stimulate digestion, it warms a cold stomach with poor digestion

---

[5]Other poison-resisting herbs: Juniper, Rue, Blessed Thistle, Elecampane, Centaury, and Garlic.

and bloating. It is helpful for cystitis after a chill. It has a warming effect on the circulation, especially cold hands and feet and so is helpful in Reynaud's and chilblains. Angelica has a strong emmenagogue action and should be avoided in pregnancy, although the tea can be drunk in a stalled labour. It is excellent for menstrual cramps and heavy, dragging pains in menstruation, which are due to cold. It is similar to the Chinese herb Dong Quai (*Angelica sinensis*) which is used extensively for women's reproductive conditions including menopause.

Emotional virtues

Angelica has a powerful, fiery energy. It is about action, initiation, giving a bit of gumption to the weak and windy. It has strong leadership energy, use for finding your voice, speaking your truth, being heard, making your case. It is a female, light-hearted warrior; a strong leader, kindly, but definitely the boss; joyful, strong, fiery, high-energy, like a firecracker. It has the quality of excitement, needing to run and dance and fly. It is especially good for people who feel stuck in a rut, who need courage for a new start or big plan, for finding power. Angelica is heady and a bit wild and so can be too strong for the ungrounded. Angelica is a joyful herb and banishes negative energy, attracts positive energy, and enhances the aura.

Magical

Angelica is a herb for leaders, use when you need energy to start or maintain a big, bold project. It supports leaders who are kindly and inclusive, in the nature of the Sun, but who can take on leadership roles when necessary. Its association with angels means Angelica is useful in any rituals to do with angelic guidance or protection. It is a powerful protector herb, used in baths to cleanse and purify.

Ritual

Angelica boosts female power. It is lovely for big gatherings, such as festivals, where massive energy, people skills, humour, and creativity are needed. Angelica has a strong action; fiery types may need only small doses to gain an effect, too much and the excess fire might be a bit hard to handle, or, alternatively, may help to power through. It is excellent for initiating a group enterprise, for getting the show on the road, and for performers, or people who need the courage to speak in public. Also, for group meetings, to give a good feeling to participants when there has been a falling out, to keep people awake and focused. Scatter it around for protection, for removing negative energy or psychic attacks, and for healing rituals.

Angelica is a constitutional remedy for cholerics, together with Rosemary and Calendula.

Eyebright *(Euphrasia officinalis)*

Herb of the Sun in Virgo, or perhaps Leo.
Hot and dry in first degree.
Part used: herb.
Chakra: solar plexus.
Culpeper virtues: restores sight, strengthens brain, heats the head.
Modern virtues: tonic, astringent, anti-inflammatory, antiseptic, anti-catarrhal.

History

Euphrasia comes from the Greek for joy (ευφροσυνη) and was the name of one of the three Graces, Euphrosyne, who was given the plant to bring joy to those suffering from poor eyesight. Gerard used powdered Eyebright herb mixed with Mace because it "comforteth the memorie" (Grieve, 1977, p. 293). Culpepper made "An Excellent Water to Clear the Sight. Take of fennel, eyebright, roses, white, celandine, vervain and rue, of each a handful, the liver of a goat chopt small, infuse them well in eyebright water, then distil them in an alembic, and you shall have a water will clear the sight beyond comparison" (Grieve, 1977, p. 293).

Modern virtues

Eyebright contains tannins, which dry up secretions from watery and inflamed eyes. Use in diseases of the sight, weakness of the eyes, ophthalmia, blepharitis, and conjunctivitis. Eyebright combines well with Calendula for inflamed and red eyes, sties, and any eye infections, with Nettle for eye irritation and itching due to hay fever and allergies. The dried herb can be mixed with Comfrey root and used to bathe and soothe irritated eyes. Eyebright may be used in warm or cold infusions. Eyebright also combines well with Witch Hazel[6] and Raspberry leaf to bathe eyes tired from reading or excessive computer use. Soak a soft cloth in a dilute tea, or bathe the eye in an eye bath. Traditionally used for bronchitis and sore throats, dried Eyebright was an ingredient in British Herbal Tobacco, which can be smoked for chronic bronchitis and colds. It may be combined with Rosemary to improve memory and strengthen the brain. Culpeper suggests steeping fresh Eyebright and fresh Rosemary in wine and leaving in the sun for thirty to forty days to make a "physical wine" (Tobyn, 1997, p. 218). I think it would be a good combination for brain fog, tiredness, and forgetfulness.

Emotional

Eyebright, as a sunny herb, is useful to banish negativity and dark thoughts. It helps to develop a more positive outlook. It improves focus and concentration and helps with memory and studying. Eyebright brings clarity; it shows the reality of a situation and helps to find a way to disarm abusers. It clears the mind and heart, especially where there is bullying or psychological abuse, as sometimes it is difficult to recognise and accept what is happening. It helps to build a protective layer if you cannot leave the situation and to deflect critical and cruel energies.

Magical

This is a herb of spiritual growth. It increases our connection with the spiritual realms through increasing psychic sensitivity and clairvoyance. Use in spells to stop bullies and abusers, particularly for children. Carry some with you. At work, have a plant on your desk or a picture on your phone to remind you that spirit is here to protect you and show you how to move forwards. For children, make a pouch with Eyebright in it and have them carry it with them. It works equally well with children who are bullies, to soften and heal them.

---

[6]But not chemist-bought Witch Hazel, which contains alcohol. Use Witch Hazel bark in decoction.

Ritual

Use in banishing rituals for abusive partners or work colleagues. Eye-bright shows you where you need to be and gives clues as to how to get there. Use to gain clarity in any situation, for scrying and clairvoyance. It helps when dealing with a hostile crowd, classroom, or workplace.

Greater Celandine *(Chelidonium majus)*

Sun in Leo.
Hot and dry in third degree.
Chakra: heart.
Part used: root and herb.
Culpeper virtues: cutting, sharp, cleansing, heats liver and head, oph-thalmic remedy.
Modern virtues: alterative, diuretic, ophthalmic, purgative.

History

Culpeper writes: "this is one of the best cures for the eyes that is". The eyes are ruled by the luminaries (Sun and Moon). Pick Greater Celan-dine when the Sun is in Leo and the Moon is in Aries. Let Leo arise (be on the Ascendant) and make an ointment. "[T]he most desperate sore eyes have been cured by this remedy only" (Culpeper, 1798, p. 116). It is called chelidonium, after the Greek χελιδων or "swallow", because it flowers when the swallows arrive in this country and dies back when they leave. Robert Macfarlane tweeted that "chelidonias" is a word meaning "swallow-bearing wind", that is, "a westerly or south-west-erly warm spring wind that accompanies (and aids) swallows on their spring migration northwards" (RobGMacfarlane, 2018). Gerard writes that Celandine sharpens the sight and reduces the film over the eyeball. Its vivid yellow colour suggests it would be useful for jaundice. The powder of the dried root, put on an aching and lose tooth, will cause it to fall out (Culpeper, 1798, p. 117).

Modern virtues

Celandine is used in jaundice as a blood purifier and mixed with a car-minative, such as Fennel or Dill, helping to cleansing the liver and gall-bladder. It can be used as a tea or hand and foot bath to cleanse the liver.

Externally, the fresh juice has been used to cure warts, but it can burn the skin, so just drop on the affected area, do not use on unblemished skin. Celandine contains alkaloids and so its long-term use should be avoided and in pregnancy, when breastfeeding, and in cases of liver disease, unless under the supervision of a practitioner.

Emotional

Used in hand and foot baths, Celandine brings the qualities of the Sun to the emotions: warmth, optimism, hope. It lifts the mood in despondency and depression. Celandine has been made into a flower essence that helps people who find communication a problem, allowing them to respond to others in a more open-hearted, clear, way.

Magical

It is used in any contest or legal confrontation, where it provides protection and helps escape from unlawful imprisonment (see maji, p. 127). Wear some next to your skin during court cases or tribunals, to argue your case well and achieve success. It brings joy, success, and happiness (all solar attributes).

Ritual

Celandine is a herb of midsummer, to celebrate the high-point of the sun's journey around the heavens, and of midwinter, to celebrate the return of the light. Meditation on its warm, yellow petals opens the heart chakra and lifts the vital spirit of both the individual and the group.

St John's Wort *(Hypericum perfoliatum)*

Sun in Leo.
Warm and moist.
Chakra: heart.
Part used: whole herb.
Culpeper virtues: expels Choler, vulnerary, opens obstructions, dissolves swellings, emmenagogue, loosening, heats joints.
Modern virtues: vulnerary, nervine, anti-inflammatory.

History

Culpeper says St John's Wort is "under the celestial lion" (Leo) and is "governed by the sun … it is a cure of wounds, hurts and bruises, it opens obstructions, dissolves swellings, closes up the lips of a wound and strengthens the parts which are weak and feeble. The seed expels choler by sympathy and congealed blood from the stomach" (Culpeper, 1798, p. 211).

Gerard writes, St John's Wort "doth make an oile the colour of bloud, which is a most precious remedy for deep wounds and those that are thorow [throughout] the body" and that the leaves "are good to be laid upon burnings, scalding and all wounds" (Woodward, 1636, p. 541).

Dioscorides observed that a decoction of the seed (taken as a drink for forty days) cured sciatica, whereas the leaves heal burns, and a decoction drives away fevers with paroxysms (Gunther, 1968, p. 536).

Modern virtues

Well-known for its use in mild and moderate depression, it is believed St John's Wort can interact with pharmaceuticals such as SSRIs, the contraceptive pill, amphetamines, and tryptophan, amongst others. For this reason, patients on pharmaceuticals should consult a qualified herbalist before taking. It can also cause photosensitivity, so sun bathing is best avoided, and, if working outdoors, cover up and use dark glasses, a cap, or an eye shade. That said, it has been used for thousands of years for melancholy and sadness, and to heal the skin of wounds, bites, burns, and nerve pain. The anti-inflammatory action in St John's Wort oil is excellent. It is a very helpful remedy in the menopause, where tiredness and low mood can be an issue, and has been used with success in the treatment of premenstrual tension for similar conditions. But again, the caveat against mixing with allopathic medicine should be respected. An excellent internal remedy for the nervous system, St John's Wort is useful for conditions affecting the nerves such as neuralgia and numbness. It combines well with Wild Lettuce for pain relief. St John's Wort may be helpful with viruses, such as the herpes virus or shingles. Mix with other nourishing nervines such as Oats or Melissa. Externally, St John's Wort is useful for varicose veins; combine with Horse Chestnut leaves or Yarrow. It has been helpful externally for sciatica and other nerve pain as an oil or ointment. Use as a diluted tincture locally on infected wounds with Daisy or in an ointment. St John's Wort is a handy first aid remedy for wounds; use freshly mashed-up leaves and flowers.

Emotional

St John's Wort is a warm, glowing herb. It feeds the emotional heart, opening and shining a light into dark corners of the psyche. It is uplifting and smooths rough edges. Due to its lightness, it is best avoided if the person is too ungrounded, or if the person is not ready to do the work but just wants a quick fix. St John's Wort is not helpful for heavy, barren, depressive feelings, as it is too harsh. Also avoid its use in volatile people who can lose a sense of reality. There is a hard edge to the plant, a cruelty and brashness, which is selfish and unsympathetic. These qualities are needed when a person is too self-sacrificing, to gather up their energies. But avoid in a fiery, selfish person, or mix with heart-centring herbs such as Rose or Melissa to keep focused on what is good and true.

Magical

Use the oil to anoint the third eye or ajna chakra, for clear-seeing, clairvoyance, obtaining visions of the future. Use to banish negative energies and negative people, or to grow courage to protect yourself from bullying and oppression. Carry it as a talisman, or use a drop of the oil on your heart chakra before you leave the house or go on a journey. Use the oil for journeying, inner or outer. St John's Wort shines a light through, like a torch, making your path clear. Use for health, strength, happiness, and for divination.

Ritual

A herb of midsummer, St John's Wort brings the intense, fiery energy of Solis the sun god. Use in midsummer gatherings as an anointing oil for merry-making, feasting, storytelling, parties, and celebrations. St John's Wort is helpful in midwinter celebrations to remember the brightest light on the darkest night.

Venus ♀

Rulerships

Venus rules Taurus and Libra and is exalted in Pisces and in fall in Virgo, in detriment in Aries and Scorpio. She is the Lesser Benefic, cold and moist, phlegmatic.

Nature

The most feminine of planets, Venus rules love, harmony, beauty, luxury, wealth, how we relate romantically, and how we enjoy ourselves. Venus likes peace, cleanliness, fun, art, dance, and all music, poetry, and adornments. Great hostesses, Venusian types are cheerful, relaxed, and unhurried. Venus likes the good things in life: nature, flowers, perfume (and all good smells, such as essential oils), fashion, good food, and pleasant company.

Physically

Venus governs how attractive a person is, which may be more than their physical appearance. There is an ease and grace about Venusian types and, as Lilly says, they are "full of amorous excitements" (Lilly, 1647, p. 74). Venus rules the hair and complexion, the reproductive organs, the kidneys.

Well dignified

Dignified, attractive, sophisticated, pleasant, sociable, networkers, hostesses, artists, dancers, musicians, fashionistas. Enjoying food and drink and loving sweets, flirtatious, coquettish, great company.

Poorly dignified

Spendthrift, gluttonous, promiscuous, lazy, greedy, party animal, superficial, hypocritical, uses looks for advancement, wastrel.

Illnesses

Diabetes, cystitis, menstrual problems, fertility, diseases of venereal origin, impotence. Culpeper writes: "Diseases under Venus are all diseases of the wombe whatsoever, as suffocation, precipitation, dislo-cation, &c. All diseases incident to the members of generation, the reins and navel, as the running of the reins, the French pox, &c. All diseases coming by inordinate love or lust, priapismus,[7] impotencey in the act of generation diabetes, &c" (Culpeper, 1651a, p. 88).

Plants

Cowslip, Rose, Mugwort, Ladies Mantle, Elderflower, Orange Blossom, Coltsfoot, Apple, Vervain, Thyme, Violet, Lily. Herbs of Venus are the most plentiful, as they are soothing, calming, restorative, gently expul-sive, and cleansing.

Miscellaneous

Venus rules Friday and the first and eighth hour after sunrise. Her friends are all the planets except Saturn. She delights in the fifth and twelfth houses.

General characteristics

Appearance: Venus shows pretty, aromatic plants, with a pleasant appearance, and often possessing a sweet smell. Culpeper says sweet smells strengthen the heart (Culpeper, 1798, p. 9).
Element: water.
Qualities: moderately cold and a little more intensely moist.
Temperament: phlegmatic.
Function: expulsion.
Organs: the breast and reproductive organs (with the Moon), kidneys (with Mars).
Virtue and realm: the procreative virtue, the feeling virtue.
Herbs in this book: Ground Ivy, Yarrow, White Dead-Nettle, Violet, Rose, Motherwort, Daisy.
Herbs in A Woman's Book of Herbs (Brooke, 2018): Coltsfoot, Cowslip, Elderflower, Lady's Mantle, Mugwort, Pennyroyal, Thyme, and Vervain.

---

[7]Interestingly Culpeper gives "impotencey in the act of generation" to Saturn (Culpeper, 1651a, p. 88), which does make sense.

Herbs in Culpeper: Apple, Beans, Lady's Bedstraw, Bugle, Clary, Mallow, Herb Robert, Periwinkle, Peaches, Plums, Cherries, Damask Rose, Wood Sage, Rocket, Self-Heal, Sorrel, Strawberries, Silverweed, Vine, Wheat, and Figs.

Daisy *(Bellis perennis)*

Venus in Cancer.
Other names: Bruise-Wort.
Part used: flower, leaves, root.
Moist 2 cold 2.
Culpeper virtues: Tempers the heat of choler, refreshes the Liver, glutinating (holds tissues together, i.e. wound-healing).
Modern virtues: vulnerary, febrifuge, hepatic, anti-inflammatory, expectorant.

History

Gerard says: "Daisies do mitigate all kinde of paines, but especially in the joints and gout, proceeding from a hot, dry humor … if they be stamped with new butter and applied … they work better if mallows are added too … a decoction of daisies is good against agues, inflammation of the liver and all other inward parts" (Woodward, 1636, p. 637). The Latin *bellus* means handsome, pretty, agreeable or neat, although Grieve suggests it is named after a dryad Belidis but gives no further information as to who she might be (Grieve, 1977, p. 247). Culpeper says Daisy is a wound herb of great respect for internal and external use, good for wounds in the chest, as an oil, plaster, ointment, or syrup. Use for mouth ulcers, sore gums and tongue, and gut pain. "[T]hey temper the heat of choler and refresheth the liver" (Culpeper, 1798, p. 151). Use with Agrimony for gout, sciatica, or numbness. The leaves applied locally help to cool hot, inflamed, and swollen parts. Use for bruises and falls. Their cooling action dries up the moist humours, which have prevented healing, the ointment soothes running eyes, inflamed wounds, or wet or weeping wounds that won't heal (Culpeper, 1798, p. 151).

Modern virtues

Daisy has been called the English Arnica, and it has the added benefit that it is safe to take internally and, of course, grows everywhere. Arnica, when cultivated, tends to lose its healing properties, unlike Daisy, which is an excellent remedy for bruising, swellings, and wounds. It can also be used as an external application in rheumatism and arthritis. Make into an infused oil or salve for scars and any wounds. It mixes well with Lavender, Yarrow and Plantain. Drink Daisy tea for old, stubborn, coughs, to dry up the lingering phlegm. Use the tea as a mouthwash for inflamed gums and mouth ulcers; the flowers are high in vitamin C, which helps their healing properties. They cool the heat of Choler and so they are useful for burns, boils, and weeping sores. Use as a strong decoction or an infused oil. A poultice of Daisy is helpful in mastitis.

Emotional

No nonsense, earthy, practical, safe, Daisy calms the imagination and brings the person back to the here and now. There are no accidents; bruises and wounds are a reminder to pay more attention, and for children to come back into their physical bodies. As a flower remedy, Daisy helps with unworldliness, otherworldliness, to ground and centre in the physical world. Use Daisy for people who have issues being in their physical bodies, and also for the childish, or childlike, who may hurt themselves unconsciously to gain attention or care, who are feeling unloved. For those who have had a long illness, it has the quality of childlike laughter, re-connecting with the light-hearted joy of children. Use it for the hard knocks of life, for feeling battered and bruised, or for old traumas and wounds, to accomplish a deep inner healing and releasing. Taken as a tea or flower remedy, Daisy is great for nightmares and general fearfulness.

Magical

For midsummer fun, Daisy is an ideal flower for celebration. Make daisy-chains and crowns. Bring innocence and joy to the festivities. It has the quality of innocence. Use in children's spells, or to call the souls of children yet to be born.

Self-care

The making of your own remedy is the ultimate self-care. Use Daisy after setbacks; physical, emotional, and mental. Make when the Moon is in Taurus or Cancer, or on a Friday (Venus) or a Monday (Moon).

To make a flower essence or remedy

Take an unused glass bowl that has been washed in running water.

Fill it full of spring water.

Collect the flower heads and gently lay them in the water so they face the sun. Try to handle them as little as possible. Situate the bowl so that the sun is reflected in the water, and leave for at least four hours, or the whole day if possible.

Pick the flower heads out one by one and pour the water into a large, brown glass jar. Add the same quantity again of brandy. The brandy will "fix" the remedy and prevent it going off.

The attitude of the maker influences the nature of the remedy. Remember that water picks up vibrations and positive and negative energies and these alter the structure of the water (Emoto, 2004).[8] Centre yourself, banish negative emotions, have a clean body and open, unconflicted mind. Make the remedy in an atmosphere of peace and loving kindness.

Take four drops of this mother essence, add it to a small dropper bottle, and top up with brandy. Shake vigorously to energise and combine the remedy. Take four drops three times a day, or as required.

Daisy is also used in baños (see p. 132).

Ritual

Daisy has the quality of innocence and playfulness. We all remember making daisy chains as small children, and how compelling it is to pick the flowers. It is used in faery magic, for the goddess Freya, and to work with the fae. Use in baby blessings, for protection, luck, and to banish fears.

Daisy is a constitutional remedy for phlegmatics, along with Violet.

Ground Ivy *(Glechoma hederacea)*

Venus possibly in an Earth sign such as Virgo.
Chakra: solar plexus, root.
Hot 2 dry 2.

---

[8]Dr Emoto photographed crystals formed in frozen water, which showed startling differences when the water had been shouted at, said loving words to, exposed to different kinds of music, etc.

Part used: herb.

Other names: Ale Hoof.

Culpeper virtues: quick, sharp, bitter, heating diuretic. Biting, cutting action. Purges the head of rheumatic humours from the brain. Vulnerary. Purges choleric from stomach and melancholic humours from the spleen. Opening, heats bowels. For internal and external wounds.

Modern virtues: bitter, diuretic, astringent, tonic, gentle stimulant, anti-inflammatory, hepatic, expectorant, anti-catarrhal, vulnerary.

History

Gerard says: "against the humming noise and ringing sound of the ears, being put into them, and for them that are hard of hearing" (Grieve, 1977, p. 443). Dioscorides writes that a decoction "is a remedy against sciatica or ache in the huckle-bone" (Grieve, 1977, p. 443). Galen said that Ground Ivy, Celandine, and Daisies, in equal quantities, mashed up with a little sugar and rose water, dropped into the eyes, "takes away all manner of inflammation, etc. yea, although the sight were well known gone" (Grieve, 1977, p. 443). Culpeper added: "this is a herb of Venus so it cures the diseases she causes by sympathy and those of Mars by antipathy … a singular herb for all inward wounds, ulcerated lungs and other parts, either by himself or boiled with other herbs for windy and choleric humours in the stomach, spleen, etc. It helps the yellow jaundice, by opening the stoppings of gall and liver and melancholy by opening the stoppings of the spleen … it is excellent to gargle any sore mouth or throat and to wash sores and ulcers; it speedily heals green wounds, being bruised and bound thereto" (Culpeper, 1798, p. 56). He also writes that the juice of Ground Ivy, Celandine and Daisy is "*a sovereign remedy for the eyes*", the "*pains, redness and watering of them*", and also that "*the juice dropped into the ears wonderfully helps the noise and ringing of them*" (Culpeper, 1798, p. 56).

Modern virtues

Ground Ivy is a remedy for the respiratory system, especially stubborn coughs and catarrh and sinus problems. It is used for tinnitus taken as a tea, and is a cold and flu remedy. As an antispasmodic it is helpful for irritating and non-productive coughs. It is useful for nervous headaches. Country people call it "gill tea" and it was sold in London for making a tea to purify the blood (Grieve, 1977, p. 376). It has been found to be helpful for alleviating period pain, taken a week before the bleeding is due. It was also used to support the kidneys in lung conditions, and is a gentle liver remedy. Ground Ivy is one of the first medicinal plants to appear in late winter and early spring, along with Nettle and Cleavers. To my mind this trio of plants appear just when our immunity is at its lowest, when we are more likely to fall prey to colds and flu. Ground Ivy has a high vitamin C content as well as being diuretic and diaphoretic and so, with Cleavers and Nettle forms an excellent tea mixture for nipping colds in the bud. Culpeper recommends it for "sores and ulcers of the privy parts" (Culpeper, 1798, p. 56) and so it is a useful addition in yoni steams (see p. 120), especially for cystitis and local irritation.

Emotional

This low-growing, humble plant has a no-nonsense type of energy, no frills, no jargon, just getting on with it. It gathers all the emotions together to sort and untangle them. Only when order has been restored can decisions be made. For people who do too much, it helps them focus and hunker down.

Magical

Ground Ivy is earthy and slow and cautious. It has the energy of the old ways, forest crone wisdom, ancient teachings. It balances and centres and puts experiences in the perspective of time and history. Tie above the crib of a fearful baby. At death, decorate the coffin, or, at the laying out, it can be buried with the body to send the person back to the ancestors and connect with their ground and root.

Ritual

For solitary practitioners. Keep on the altar in springtime, from Candlemas to the spring equinox, to contemplate the lowly, the humble, the early bird. Ground Ivy is a reminder to keep it simple and uncomplicated. It contains the wise, old, fairy wisdom of the ages. Use as a focus for meditation, for beauty, simplicity, order, structure, peace, and wisdom.

Motherwort *(Leonurus cardiaca)*

Venus in Leo.
Part used: the herb.
Hot 2 dry 2.
Chakra: heart.
Culpeper virtues: cleansing, binding, purges melancholy from the heart, dries up cold humours.
Modern virtues: diaphoretic, antispasmodic, nervine, emmenagogue.

History

Culpeper gives it to Venus in Leo, and says there "is no better herb to drive away melancholy vapours from the heart, to strengthen it and make the mind cheerful, blithe and merry" (Culpeper, 1798, p. 253) taken as a syrup of conserve. He says it warms and dries up cold humours, digesting and dispersing those that are settled in the veins, joints, and sinews of the body, helping cramps and convulsions. The Latins call it *cordiaca*, and "it cleanseth the chest of cold phlegm" (Culpeper, 1798, p. 253). Gerard uses it "against infirmities of the heart … it is good for them that are in hard travail with childe" (Woodward, 1636, p. 705).

Modern virtues

Motherwort is specific for menopause, hot flushes, palpitations, poor circulation, hypertension, anxiety, and depression and insomnia. It can be used as a general tonic in menopause with Nettle and Cleavers. For insomnia, Motherwort mixes well with Limeflower, for sweats, with Red Clover, and for weakness with Nettle and Melissa. It is heating and stimulating for sluggish, cold conditions. However, avoid where there is heavy bleeding as it may exacerbate the problem. It can be used for high blood pressure as a tea or tincture. It also mixes well with Hawthorn, Cleavers, Nettle, and Dandelion herb.

Emotional

Motherwort has a light, bouncy, happy, laughing energy, and so use it for people who are suffering from tiredness, heart-weariness, and where there is weakness, indecision, lack of willpower. It is useful after extreme emotional shock; its warm, motherly energy brings feelings of safety and calm. For extreme stress, such as exams or being judged in some way, it brings a deep, warm, sedative sleep, like a mother tucking you up in bed. It has a no-nonsense, matter-of-fact, practical, grounded, secure, safe, and sensible energy. Motherwort is uncomplicated, good, straightforward, and loving, like a country mother. Use in menopause when the body feels out of control, bringing stability, calm, and security.

Magical

Motherwort is a charming, mature woman, confident in her own power, standing in power, standing in blood. Use it for Red Tent matters, the blood and guts of menstruation, for lost periods, for heavy, dragging, bloody periods, and to say farewell to periods, or for a lost pregnancy. Working on the heart chakra, it gives courage to cross divides, enter new phases, and on the womb chakra it gives calm and firmness in the face of danger and threat, by building a matrix of power from deep within. Drink it as a tea from the dark moon to the full, for releasing people, places, and events.

Ritual

Use for birthing rituals, crone rituals, when we let go of the blood and remove the cloak of fertility and put on the mantle of crone wisdom and power, of deeper, ancient mysteries, which in turn provide protection, wisdom, and guidance for younger women. Drink during periods to release the blood and perhaps the hope of conception, while building womb wisdom and strength.

Rose *(Rosa spp.)*

Red Rose, Jupiter. Damask Rose, Venus. White Rose, Moon.
Cold 1, dry 1 (White Rose, more so).
Parts used: flower, buds, and petals.
Chakra: heart.
Culpeper virtues: strengthens animal and vital virtues, astringent. Cools head, lungs, heart, and stomach. Red Rose is binding and mitigates heart pain. Damask Rose purges Choler, cools the head, heart, and lungs, and is cleansing.
Modern virtues: nervine, cardiac tonic, astringent, aphrodisiac.

History

Gerard writes that the distilled water of White Rose "strengthens the heart and refreshes the spirits and likewise for all things that need a gentle cooling ... the syrup doth moisten and coole, in hot burning fevers" (Woodward, 1636, p. 1263). Red Roses "strengthen the heart and helpe the trembling and beating thereof ... they give strength to the liver and kidneys and weak entrails ... they dry and comfort a weak stomach ... the honey of rose (rose melrosarum)—is good for wounds, ulcers and such things that need to be cleaned and dried ... the oyle doth mittgiate all kinds of heat' (Woodward, 1636, p. 1263). He recommends the syrup of roses as a "gentle loosening medicine carrying downwards choleric humors, opening the stoppings of the liver" (Woodward, 1636, p. 1263). He recommends the conserve of Rose (a pound of roses and four pounds of sugar, boiled together until the roses lose their colour) to strengthen the heart, and for shaking and trembling. Culpeper writes: "The electuary is purging and is good in hot fevers, jaundice and joint aches ... it cools the blood and heat in the liver" (Culpeper, 1798, p. 320). Culpeper writes that Red Rose strengthens the retentive faculty and mitigates pains from the heart, assuages inflammation, and procures rest and sleep. The juice purges the body of Phlegm and Choler. It is good in hot fevers, for pains in the head from choleric humours, and for jaundice and joint aches from heat. The syrup strengthens the stomach, cools the liver, comforts the heart, resisting infection. Honey of roses is good in gargles and lotions, for the mouth and throat. A syrup of damask purges Choler; a compound syrup works on Melancholy humours; while Rose honey is opening and purging for phlegmatic conditions.

Modern virtues

Rosewater is an excellent remedy for cooling inflamed skin, eyes, spots and blemishes, rashes. It is cooling for headaches caused by heat, and, taken as a tea with Motherwort, for menstrual pain and headache. Use Rosewater as a mouthwash for dry mouth and ulcers as side effects of radio and chemotherapy. Rose tea soothes sore throats and tonsillitis. It makes a lovely douche, mixed with a little Marigold or Myrrh, for thrush, and to cool down cystitis. Rose nourishes and replenishes the vital spirit through its action on the heart, and so it is helpful to put in mixtures for the circulatory system. It is an excellent remedy for yoni steams (p. 120) and also helpful to put in baños (p. 132) and maji (p. 127).

Emotional

Rose is an excellent heart remedy following shock, trauma, heartbreak, and all kinds of depression and anxiety. It cools agitation and restlessness, gives hope and space, and helps to drive out dark, negative feelings such as suspicion, cynicism, bitterness, and anger. Rose brings a feeling of love, wellbeing, peace, and happiness.

Magical

The association of roses with love and luxury is no coincidence. Rose opens the heart, heals the heart chakra, and removes obstacles to connection and intimacy. Clearly, they would be used in love potions, which have at their heart the self-love and self-acceptance which is prerequisite to the love of others. Baths with Rose petals, essential oils of Rose, Rose massage oils, Rose water, Rose honey: the possibilities are endless. Rose is a glorious, indulgent, gently warming, life-affirming and heart-protecting remedy. Use especially fresh roses. Rose can be used to heal sexual trauma, birth trauma, and bullying trauma by cleansing the energetic memory of the abuse. Rose cleanses the aura like a shower or cloud of pink, golden light. It invokes the blue cloak of the Great Mother; knowledge that in times of trauma we can call on the womb threads of our foremothers and our daughters-to-be, for we exist in a continuum of all women, everywhere, and at all times, to heal us and make us strong enough to resist the death machine of patriarchy in whatever way we have chosen this lifetime, and the knowledge that to resist with love is the most subversive, revolutionary action. Add to warrior mixtures to keep the heart open, such as maji (p. 127) and also baños (see p. 132).

Ritual

Rose is used in handfasting rituals, rose petals scattered on bedding, on blankets, used in wreaths and put in the hair. Rosewater is used on the body and in food, also to nourish the heart and to evoke love and passion. Due to its volatile nature, Rose is great for steaming, to release the scented oils and transfer the magical effects directly into the body.

Yoni steaming[9]

An easy way to do a steam is get a large glass bowl and fill it full of boiling spring water, adding scented and magical plants, chosen according to the effect you wish to create. Then crouch or squat or do child's pose, allowing the scented steam to be absorbed by your yoni. If you have an old chair where the seat has broken, you can put this above the bowl. It can also be placed in the bath tub: squat over the bowl holding the sides of the bath. Whichever method you chose, pick a time when you won't be disturbed for at least thirty minutes. Full moons are good for letting go of energies, new moons for bringing in the new.

You could include: Rose, for love; Marigold and Mugwort, to cleanse and disperse energies; Yarrow, to reclaim your power; Melissa, to heal trauma; and White Dead-Nettle, for restoring purity. The possibilities are endless and the delights without limit!

Violet *(Viola odorata)*

Venus.
Cold 1 Moist 2.
Part used: leaves and flowers.
Chakra: heart, crown.
Culpeper virtues: cleansing, cooling, cordial, purges Choler. Cools head, lungs, heart, and stomach. Moistens heart, mollifying (softening). Modern virtues: lymphatic, blood cleanser, anti-tussive, demulcent, expectorant.

History

Violet is one of the four cordial flowers[10] and cools the heat of the heart when excited by Choler, caused by anger, stress, and excess physical

---

[9]This idea for yoni steams came from Sarah Smith on an online herbal forum, where she recommended it for "exorcising the ghosts of boyfriends past" (private communication with herbalist Sarah Smith).
[10]The others are Borage, Rose, and Viper's Bugloss.

activity. Culpeper recommends Violet for a dry stomach, and as a syrup when there is heartburn or excess acid. Violet is cooling for Choler in the liver where there is inflammation; for hot, itchy skin, as in eczema; for constipation due to dryness; and for swollen veins or varicosities. Violet is also one of the five emollient herbs.[11] Violet cools any heat, internally or externally. It cures headache due to insomnia, mixed with oil of Rose. The leaves purge choleric humours and assuage heat. The flowers are used for quinsy (Culpeper, 1798, p. 381).

Gerard recommends Violet as cooling for all inflammations, especially the sides and lungs, hoarseness in the chest, and ruggedness of the windpipes and jaws. "Violet sugar comforts the heart and other inward parts and allays the extreme heat of the liver, kidneys and bladder ... it mitigates the sharpness of choler ... the oile doth provoke sleep which is hindered by a hot and dry distemper" (Woodward, 1636, p. 852).

Culpeper gives violets to Venus and says they "have a mild nature" and are "in no way harmful" (Culpeper, 1798, p. 381). They are cold and moist and cool heat and distemper. He uses them for inflamed eyes and hot swellings. Violet water purges choleric humours and assuages heat.

Dioscorides writes that Violet has "a cooling faculty" (Gunther, 1968, p. 513) and that the flowers, when drunk, help the inflammation of the eyes.

Modern virtues

As they are slightly cooling and moistening, violets are excellent for anxiety and anger and insomnia due to overheating. They cool and soothe the mind, calm fears, allow the brain to shut down for sleep. Use Violet tea or Violet water for headache due to heat and tension. Violet is such a gentle remedy (although powerful) it can be included in sleep mixes for infants, children, and the elderly. It works well mixed with Chamomile, Limeflower and Lavender. Violet soothes a dry, irritating cough, and works especially well with Marshmallow and Liquorice. Its demulcent action helps to release trapped Phlegm, calms the airways, and facilitates expectoration. It is a lymphatic stimulant, so is helpful after glandular fever, influenza, and other viral conditions where the immune system needs a boost, and is traditionally used in cancer treatments. Locally, its cooling action soothes heated and irritated skin in

---

[11]The others are Marshmallow, Pellitory, Linseed, and Fenugreek.

cases such as dermatitis and eczema (use as a tea or gel). Violet is also used as a poultice to dissolve hard swellings, and can be used as a tea and poultice for mastitis. Grieve reports syrup of Violet can be used as a laxative for infants (Grieve, 1977, p. 838). Along with Cleavers and Nettles (see Brooke, 2018), Violet is one of the first early spring flowers; it often comes out around Imbolc (2 February). I use all three herbs in a mix for that festival, and as an early spring tonic to banish the February blues. Cleavers unplugs the lymphatic system and gets the fluids moving, Nettle kickstarts the kidneys, excretes urine, and heats up the body, as well as adding much-needed minerals. Violet adds a bit of sunshine and light and relaxation during the coldest, wettest, most miserable months.

Emotional

Working on the heart chakra, Violet will sweeten sour hearts, and warm cold hearts. It has a warm, maternal energy, protective, nurturing, giving a feeling of safety when fearful and fretting. Use Violet to find clarity and resolve, and to banish dark, hidden worries. It lightens soggy energy. Mix with Rose or Marigold or Hawthorn flowers to brighten and lighten a heavy load. Violet calms the temper, brings sleep and prophetic dreams and visions. Water Violet is a Bach flower remedy, for people who prefer to be alone and may be seen as stand-offish or cold by others. Often these are creative or nature-loving people who are happy with their own company, but they may suffer from loneliness.

Magical

Violet has the quality of sunlight on water: clear and cool, smoothing sharp, jagged edges. Use for aura cleansing, as a tea or flower water. Violet also works on the crown chakra; use it to brush up your "halo", bringing bright, clear, and clean spiritual energy into your life. It encourages self-loving kindness for the young and the elderly, to banish grief or disappointment or old hurts that need to be forgiven; loss buried in a cold body. Ideal for inflexible, rigid people, emotionally dogmatic types. Use the leaf to have dreams of the future: drink or put in a bath before bed. Use with Lavender for love spells, and in spells to change your luck and for good fortune.

Ritual

Violet is an excellent herb for rituals and celebrations, such as hand-fastings and naming ceremonies. It gives joy, laughter, and a sense of community. Take as a tea for happy group meetings. It goes well at Beltane and Midsummer celebrations with their joyful, female energies. It encourages creativity, peace, and tranquillity.

Violet is a constitutional remedy for phlegmatics, together with Daisy.

White Dead-Nettle *(Lamium album)*

Venus.
Hot 3 dry 3.
Chakra: heart, ajna.
Other names: Archangel, Bee Nettle.
Part used: herb.
Culpeper virtue: drying and binding, helps the retentive faculty, heats throat and womb.
Modern virtue: astringent, anti-spasmodic, diuretic, anti-inflammatory.

History

It is called Archangel because traditionally it comes into flower on the day of Archangel Michael (8 May old calendar, now 27 April). It is also known as Bee Nettle, as it attracts bees into a garden. The generic name, *Lamium*, comes from λαιμος (Greek, "throat"), which may refer to the shape of the flower or its properties. Gerard says: "the flowers baked with sugar, and distilled water of them, is used to make the heart merry … refreshes the Vital Spirits" (Woodward, 1636, p. 705). Culpepper says Archangel is "somewhat hotter and drier than stinging nettles and is used with better success to stop hardness of the Spleen using a decoction of the herb in wine. The flowers if preserved and conserved stay the whites [leucorrhoea]" (Culpeper, 1798, p. 65). He agrees with Gerard that Archangel "makes the heart merry, drives away melancholy, quickens the spirits" (Culpeper, 1798, p. 65). He recommended it to relieve hardness of the spleen (the seat of Melancholy) if taken as a decoction in wine.

Modern virtues

White Dead-Nettle has an astringent nature and therefore is drying for haemorrhages, discharges and cold, damp, phlegmatic conditions. The anti-spasmodic action helps with period pains and has been used successfully in Pelvic Inflammatory Disease with Calendula, Echinacea, and Myrrh. I have used it successfully for thrush and discharges. As an astringent it is useful for chronic cystitis or the cystitis/thrush merry-go-round that occurs with antibiotics. White Dead-Nettle purifies the blood in skin conditions such as eczema and rashes, taken as a decoction. Locally, the tincture dabbed on a cut will staunch the blood-flow. It can also be used as a poultice or salve for wounds, bruises, pains in the joints and muscles, and as an astringent for varicose veins and haemorrhoids.

Emotional

I give it to Venus in Leo because it has a gentle warmth. It works on the ajna chakra and the heart, and has lightening qualities of Fire with Earth. It has a youthful, feminine, light, airy, clear, fresh, spring-time, energy. It allows us to embrace the world with arms open wide; it has expansive feeling and the optimism and energy of youth. White Dead-Nettle is happiness, meadows, sunlight, laughing, pleasure, gently warming. It evokes young sexuality (menarche rituals), female power, being awestruck at young female beauty, recalling innocence, purity, and lightness. Use it for temporary dark states, when connection to these energies has been lost, to find the clarity and light-heartedness again. Use also when suffering from long-term gynaecological problems, to joyfully re-connect with your fertile, amazing, female body.

Magical

Use it to connect with real female power and banish negative, hate-filled, patriarchal images of womanhood. Use it in yoni steam (p. 120), or in baths (use the flower heads and breathe deeply their honied perfume). Use for scrying and clairvoyance; it gives clear-sightedness, direction, and uncomplicated answers. White Dead-Nettle is one of my favourite herbs for a baño (see p. 132). Use for protection, healing, and to block bad energy.

Ritual

Use in rituals to recall and restore innocence and purity and real feminine power: spring equinox, Beltane, menarche, after childbirth, or after any trauma or setback. With its soaring, releasing energy, White Dead-Nettle can also be used at the end of life, to move on, let go of a sick or aged body, and move towards the light with full-heartedness and joy.

Yarrow *(Achillea millefolium)*

Venus.
Cold 1 dry 1.
Part used: whole herb.
Other names: Milfoil, Nose Bleed.
Culpeper virtues: cools kidney and bladder. Astringent, healing, strengthens retentive virtue, binding.
Modern virtues: bitter, diaphoretic, diuretic, hepatic, anti-coagulant, relaxant, circulatory, anti-spasmodic, astringent.

History

Other names for Yarrow indicate its actions: Milfoil, Old Man's Pepper, Nose Bleed, Knight's Milfoil, Soldier's Woundwort, Devil's Nettle: Yarrow was used as a wound healer, applied as a salve. Gerard wrote that Achilles, the Greek warrior, used it to staunch the wounds of his soldiers. Others suggest it was discovered by the same Achilles, who was a pupil of Chiron, the healer, which is why the genus is known as *Achillea*. Its specific name *millefolium* reflects Yarrow's feathery leaves (Grieve, 1977, p. 864). It was called Nose Bleed as the leaves can both stop bleeding (the leaf rolled up, inserted into the nose) and induce nose bleeds for the relief of headache. Gerard writes that it is cleansing, "cold and binding ... the leaves do close up wounds and keep them from inflammation ... it stauncheth blood in any part of the body ... put into bathes for women to sit in it ... the green leaves chewed for toothache" (Woodward, 1636, p. 1073). Culpeper says that because it is drying and binding it cures wounds, stops inflammation, and stops "the bloody flux" (dysentery). He recommends it as an ointment for green wounds, ulcers, and fistulas, especially where there is moisture (discharges). He recommends it to strengthen the retentive faculty of the stomach, where there is vomiting. Finally, he suggests chewing the leaves for toothache (Culpeper, 1798, p. 389).

Modern virtues

As a tea, Yarrow is excellent for severe colds and fevers as it brings on a big sweat to ease the infection out. Sweetened with a little honey or sugar, use for children's fevers such as chickenpox and measles. It is also great for period pains due to pelvic congestion, as well as heavy bleeding and menopausal symptoms such as sweats. As a tea or tincture use for circulatory problems associated with liver congestion, such as varicose veins. It is a local vaso-dilator for thrombosis. It is a great herb for a high blood-pressure mix, with Hawthorn berries, Limeflower and Motherwort. Yarrow is anti-inflammatory and can help with arthritis, especially where there is poor circulation or liver issues. The fresh herb can be used as a wound healer and to stop bleeding. Dioscorides agrees: "excellent for an excessive discharge of blood, and old and new ulcers" (Gunther, 1968, p. 651).

Emotional

Although given to Venus, I feel that Yarrow has strong martial properties. Perhaps it is a herb of Venus in Aries or Scorpio. It is heady, rising, connecting the head and the heart, but is a herb of the slow step, not dancing like White Dead-Nettle nor plodding like Black Horehound, but marching with a firm, steady, stride, neither earth-bound nor soaring, but centred in its power. Yarrow is not so much a warrior as an activist, a fighter for justice, a lawyer or campaigner; she is less for direct action, as this is too messy, but more a campaigner who uses her head and heart. Yarrow has a cool intellect, a wry humour, but is also implacable. She focuses the mind, ends chatter, uses her briefcase and intelligence as armour. She has a no-nonsense energy and a honied tongue that offers protection via the intellect or speech. Yarrow uses patriarchy's own laws to fight it with humour and grace (Venus), but she is implacable, a warrior of the mind, laughing at their stupidity, incompetence, tying them in knots, honey on the razor's edge.

Use in menarche to put some steel into a young girl's psyche, laughing at the fools, but having your weapons ready. Yarrow gives backbone.

Magical

Yarrow helps you to put on your battle armour, to fight injustice, to stand and be counted. It gives courage, perseverance, hope. It is known as the Witch's Herb. It promotes self-confidence. To ward off fear wear it on your body. It calms anger and focuses it and re-directs it. It is useful for binding emotional and psychic wounds. A magical preparation, "maji", can be used when facing enemies. Rub it on your arms, the back of your neck and your face and forehead. It contains alcohol, and so avoid the eyes as they will sting.

Maji[12]

You can use a variety of herbs, depending on the results you are looking for. Check the magical uses in this book and *A Woman's Book of Herbs* (Brooke, 2018) to get the best combination of energies. Examples include: for warrior-like activity, Yarrow, Milk Thistle, Nettle or Nettle seeds; for focus, White Willow bark; to keep the heart engaged (so you don't get lost in rage), Rose, Melissa, Rosemary; to keep grounded, roots, Hyssop; for dragon energy and courage, Thyme; for empowerment after attack, Comfrey.

Prepare at the full moon for more potency. Take your herbs (fresh is better, but dried will work), put them in a big pot or big pestle and mortar (like the African ones), and mash them up together with a little alcohol. Add essential oils and Bach Flower Remedies as required.

Traditionally, the mixing and pounding is done by each member, who sings a ritual song to put their energy into the mixture. This creates a group energy, which makes resistance and cohesion so much stronger.

The mix should be reduced to small pieces, so they can fit inside a bottle of 100ml or so. Pour in enough alcohol (such as vodka, or cider vinegar if you don't want alcohol) to cover, and leave about a handswidth above the mash. Mix thoroughly, add more liquid to make it run, like a thick tincture. Decant into bottles and carry with you. Apply as required to power points, such as the heart, the back of the neck, the brows, the arms and hands and face.

---

[12]Maji is the name for a herbal preparation made in Gaga, Petro Voodoo practised in the Dominican Republic and elsewhere by the African diaspora. It consists of 101 magical herbs, which are pounded in a giant wooden pestle and mortar, steeped in rum, and then used as protection during dances in the streets from Good Friday to Easter Sunday.

Ritual

For clarity use Yarrow in scrying, focusing. Drink the tea or burn as incense for clarity like a big sword cutting through the confusion. Use to cut the cords with other people, events, or places. On a fire moon or Tuesday (Mars) drink the tea and burn the incense, close they eyes and visualise the etheric body and, with a great iron sword or knives or a dagger, cut any chains which bind you to the past. Remove any knives or daggers others have left in you. Drink the tea for a week afterwards to heal the wounds. The name Devil's Nettle, reflects its use in divination and spells. Dried yarrow stalks were used for divination with the *I Ching*.

Mercury ☿

Rulerships

Mercury rules Gemini and Virgo and is in detriment in Sagittarius and in fall in Pisces. He is neither masculine nor feminine as Mercury takes on the nature of any planet it aspects.

Nature

A melancholy planet, cold and dry, but because of its mutable nature if Mercury aspects a benefic planet like Jupiter it has a positive action. Conversely, if it aspects a malefic such as Mars, it has a negative action. Mercury is said to rule animal spirit. Mercury is the trickster. Lilly says: "he is author of subtilty, tricks, devices, perjury etc." (Lilly, 1647, p. 77). Hermes in mythology was the only god who could travel between all three realms: heaven, earth, and the underworld. Mercury brings messages from spirit and from the unconscious, translating both for humankind.

Physically

A strong Mercury gives a slim, neat, compact body. The person has a timeless quality, and they often look younger than their years, sometimes surprisingly so. They often have beautiful or delicate hands and feet. Quick-witted, they move and talk rapidly, and dislike sitting and waiting. Mercury rules the mind, respiration, sight, speech, the arms and hands and the nervous system.

Well dignified

Like the other melancholic planets, a strong Mercury will give great intelligence although it will be of a different kind from Saturn's orderliness. Here, the mind is rapid, full of bright ideas, making connections, pulling inspiration (from the Latin *inspirare*, "to breathe in") from the heavens and from the unconscious. Mercury gives fluid speech, a great arguer and debater. A strong Mercury is often found in politicians and teachers and communicators of all types. A lover of technology and logic, a strong Mercury shows charming, bubbly, interested, open-minded, funny people. Mercury gives great travellers, people who are interested in new experiences, also salesmen, merchants, writers, bloggers, journalists, teachers, all showing Mercury's facility with language and languages.

Poorly dignified

A weak Mercury shows liars, thieves, con-men, disputatiousness, slander, gossip, muck-raking, boasting, nosiness, foolishness, immaturity, cruel practical jokers, incautiousness, fickleness, unreliability, "constant in nothing but idle words and bragging" (Lilly, 1647, p. 78).

Illnesses

Stuttering, speech defects, dizziness, fainting, disease of the hands and feet, memory loss, dementia, hysteria, anxiety, frenzy, hoarseness, dry cough, mania, wind and bloating, dyspraxia, dyslexia. Culpeper writes: "Under Mercury are almost all the diseases of the braine, as vertigo's, madnesse, &c. all diseases of the lungs, as Asthma, Phthisicks, &c. All imperfections of the Tongue, as stammering, lisping, &c. Hoarsnesse, coughs, snuffling in the nose: all defects of the memory (with Saturn) … stopping of the head, dumbnesse, folly and simplicity (the Epidemicall diseases of the time) and whatsoever hurts the intellectuall faculty" (Culpeper, 1651a, p. 88).

Herbs

This book: Honeysuckle, Jack by the Hedge, Oats, White Horehound.

A Woman's Book of Herbs (Brooke, 2018): Elecampane, Lavender, Fennel, Liquorice, and Valerian.

Miscellaneous

Mercury rules Wednesday and the first and eighth hours after sunrise. Mercury is happy in the ascendant and the sixth houses. His friends are Jupiter, Venus, and Saturn, and his enemies are all the other planets. Mercury rules short trips and modes of transport, such as bicycles.

General characteristics

Appearance: plants ruled by mercury are multicoloured; Culpeper describes them as *codded* ("with pouches or sacks") and *arenary* ("sand-like", perhaps growing on sandy soil).

Element: Earth.

Qualities: Mercury is a mutable planet, dry with the dry, moist with the moist, warm with the warm, and cool with the cool; it is affected by whatever is nearby.

Temperament: melancholic.

Function: retention.

Organ: nerves and lungs.

Realm and virtue: animal virtue, the nerves, thought, intellect.

Sense: common sense, imagination.

Herbs in this book: (see above).

Herbs in *A Woman's Book of Herbs* (Brooke, 2018): (see above).

Herbs in Culpeper: Carrot, Caraway, Dill, Hazelnut, Marjoram, Mulberries, Parsley, Pellitory of the Wall, Samphire, Summer Savory, Southernwood.

Honeysuckle *(Lonicera caprifolium)*

Mercury in Cancer.

Part used: the flowers.

Other names: Woodbine.

Hot 3, dry 3.

Culpeper virtues: purges Melancholy and Phlegm, loosening.
Modern virtues: cutaneous tonic, vulnerary, diuretic, sudorific, anti-spasmodic, anodyne, nervine, expectorant, laxative.

History

A decoction of the flowers or the flower water is said to be anti-spasmodic and is an excellent remedy for headache and anxiety. Gerard recommends steeping the flowers in oil in direct sunlight for a several weeks, and then using for "benumbed and very cold bodies … a syrup of the flowers is good … against diseases of the lungs and spleen that is stopped … [W]ater of honeysuckle is good against the soreness of the throat" (Woodward, 1636, p. 891). Culpeper gives honeysuckle to Mercury in Cancer, while suggesting it is not a foe to Leo. He recommends the conserve of the flowers as a cure for asthma and to take away the *"evil of the spleen"* (Culpeper, 1798, p. 387), i.e. melancholy. It provokes the urine and ensures a speedy delivery in childbirth. He recommends it for cramps, convulsions, and palsies, as well as *"griefs from cold or stoppings"* (Culpeper, 1798, p. 387), i.e. phlegmatic and melancholic causes. He recommends it made into an ointment for freckles and sunburn. Interestingly, Dioscorides suggests that a "decoction taken for thirty-seven days is said to make men unfit for generation" (Gunther, 1968, p. 555).

Modern virtues

Honeysuckle is used in Traditional Chinese Medicine to clear heat and poisons from the body. It is useful for digestive complaints like diarrhoea and cramping. As a respiratory herb, it is helpful for viral and bacterial infections such as flu, viruses, and coughs. It combines well with Cowslip for coughs and demulcent remedies like Marshmallow for asthma. It is a febrifuge and lowers temperature in infections. It calms headaches caused by heat. Used externally it warms the extremities, so is used for Reynaud's syndrome or chilblains.

Emotional

Honeysuckle is one of the Bach Flower remedies, used for homesickness, longing for the past, bereavement, and any loss causing hopelessness and the feeling that the person will not have the same happiness again. Use where the patient shows wistfulness and nostalgia and an unwillingness to be in the present. Use for prosperity, luck, peace, success, and drawing money to you quickly. It increases persuasiveness, confidence, and sharpens the intuition.

Magical

Use Honeysuckle to make a baño.[13] Pick a sunny day and start in the morning. Full moon is a good time. Take several handfuls of fresh Violet flowers, Rose petals, Mugwort, White Dead-Nettle, Lavender, Motherwort, or any other mixture of herbs depending on the effect you are looking for. Put in a large bowl (washing-up bowl size) three quarters full of fresh spring water. Tear the leaves and flowers until they are all mixed together into a mush and swish around in the water.

Situate the bowl so the sun is reflected in the water. Keep pets and children away. Every hour or so, check the sun is still reflected in the water; move the bowl to follow the sun.

Just before sunset, take the bowl and strain the liquid into a large jug. Have a shower and dry yourself, and then massage in some body oil. Then pour the baño over your head.

Lie down in a warm place and sleep or sit and meditate.

Your dreams or meditations may answer any question you need answering.

Baños are best done three days in a row.

Classically, baños are done to attract a partner, but they can also be used for courage, insight, finding a home, jobs, and health. Look up the emotional, magical, and ritual uses of the herbs and chose ones that fit your purpose.

Baños can be done at night, with the reflected light of the moon. Willow and other watery, witchy herbs would be ideal. Again, look at the virtues of the plants to pick your mixture.

---

[13]I learned to make baños from the Haitian wise women at the botanica in the Mercado Modelo in Santo Domingo. They suggest doing them on Tuesdays and Fridays for three days, Tuesdays and Fridays falling on the thirteenth of the month being especially favourable. Of course, the sun shines most of the time, in the Caribbean; in the UK, we have to pick our days when we can.

Ritual

Use Honeysuckle when in full flower for summertime, full-moon rituals, blessings, naming ceremonies and handfastings. Because of its warm, bountiful nature it will bring a feeling of peace and wellbeing to any gathering, especially where children are present, or where love and nurturing are the themes. It develops clairvoyance; use the infused oil to understand dreams and to perform astral travelling. Honeysuckle is traditionally used in love potions, spells, and rituals. Loving yourself is the first step to finding a partner.

Honeysuckle is a constitutional remedy for melancholics, together with Comfrey.

Jack by the Hedge *(Sisymbrium alliaria [Alliaria petiolata])*

Mercury.
Hot 4 dry 4.
Other names: Sauce Alone, Garlic Mustard.
Part used: herb and seed.
Culpeper virtues: digests Phlegm, warms the stomach, digestive, expectorant.
Modern virtues: sudorific, antiseptic, diuretic, stimulant, bitter.

History

Traditionally used to make a sauce for fish and other cold, damp foods, it is one of the oldest spices used in cooking. It has been found in graves in the Baltic, dated 4100-3740 BCE. It can be used in salads where its warmth aids digestion. It is a great herb for spicy pesto and pasta sauces. It is one of the early flowering green herbs which are high in vitamin C, excellent as a blood cleaner for spring fasts.

Culpeper virtues

The juice boiled with honey is excellent for coughs to shift thick phlegm and aid in expectoration of thick mucus. The crushed seed boiled in wine is a good remedy for wind colic and the stone, and for menstrual problems, drunk and applied locally (the seed put into a cloth and applied when warm). The green leaves are held to heal ulcers in the legs (Culpeper, 1798, p. 290).

Modern virtues

The juice of the leaves taken alone or boiled into a syrup is helpful in oedema. It is used externally for infected wounds and ulcers. It is useful for warming a slow digestion, and as a cough remedy for long-standing, hard-to-shift conditions. Use after long, debilitating illnesses or emotional suffering, where the immune system is compromised and the person is suffering from continual colds, and other cold, damp, conditions. It can be incorporated into hot rubs for muscle aches with other stimulating herbs, or for chest rubs. However, as a member of the mustard family, Jack by the Hedge can be an irritant to the skin, and is best avoided in children and with delicate or reactive skin.

Emotional

The fiery nature of the plant helps in grief and slow, sad emotions of long duration. It benefits sensitive and gentle people where strength and perseverance are needed. It brings fire into the heart, to build strength and find joy again. Use in adolescence, connecting to the divine masculine.

Magical

Masculine initiation rites, vision quests, epitomised by the Green Man, the embodiment of virile, potent, playful masculinity rooted in nature. Also, he represents Hern the Hunter, masculine god of the chase and the wild. The embodiment of the wild man, the provider.

Ritual

Drink at Beltane, to celebrate and embody the Green Man. Season hunted meat and fish with the herb. Drink to celebrate Hern during the Hunter's Moon at the autumn equinox.

Jack in the Hedge is a constitutional remedy for choleric temperament.

Oats *(Avena sativa)*

Mercury.
Cold 1 dry 1.
Part used: tops of the oats, harvested while they are in the milky stage.
Culpeper virtues: healing, soothing, nutritive, dissolving.
Modern virtues: nervous system trophorestorative, aphrodisiac.

History

Culpeper suggests mainly external uses for Oats; for example, mixed with salt and heated to as hot as can be endured, it is used as a poultice for colic in the belly and pains in the side. Mixed with Bay oil it is helpful as a poultice for hard swellings. Oats boiled in milk were used to stop diarrhoea (this might be a good remedy for children or the elderly, substituting nut milks as required). This same remedy, sweetened with sugar, will also help to soothe a hot, dry, irritating cough (Culpeper, 1798, p. 272).

Modern virtues

Oats are rich in B vitamins, calcium, and magnesium, which strengthen and nourish the nervous system. Oats are food for the nervous system, and are the go-to remedy for nervous exhaustion, debility, insomnia, anxiety, and lack of focus and concentration. After shock or heartbreak, oats can re-build shattered peace of mind and nourish and restore normal nervous responses. Strong but gentle, they can be taken by children and the elderly to gradually build up strength and resilience in the nervous system. Use especially for fearful children and adults, who are light sleepers and experience poor-quality, interrupted sleep. Use for longstanding generalised anxiety or feelings of being overwhelmed. Oats gently restore vitality and nervous health, but bring on many deep sleeps before that happens. Use in baths for soothing fractious babies and children with eczema, or after a long, hard, day. Oats may work on the endocrine system to restore libido after long illness or trauma. The phrase "sowing your wild oats" suggests its use as an aphrodisiac and sexual stimulant. Post-childbirth, Oats can help to grow reserves of energy and bring feelings of peace and wellbeing after medical misadventures. Oats restore a sense of autonomy and agency to traumatised reproductive systems.

Emotional

Oats are soothing and strong. They go deep to the core, calming, centring and slowing down, like a cool hand across a feverish brow. Use for nervous and fearful children who perhaps are not well-grounded in the material world and hear messages from spirit and are afraid. Use for nightmares and hauntings in children and adults, and to give strength and respite from stress due to bullying and mistreatment. Oats help to centre and re-orientate, to bring fractured and split-apart emotions together. Oats make soothing baths to provide the strength to start healing and to begin self-nourishing and self-care. After being in a toxic environment, an oat bath or tea or strong decoction helps to soothe and heal and nourish the body and re-group the emotions. For shock, exhaustion, and after trauma, use Oats to revitalise. They are calming rather than grounding.

Wild Oats are a Bach Flower remedy, and one of the first I saw work spectacularly when I was a newly qualified herbalist. It is the remedy that finds your path in life. Frequently, I added it to the mix for patients who did not know what to do, or were at a crossroads and found it hard to make a choice as to their next move. Without fail they would return in a fortnight, clear and calm, decided upon their path, and often their physical symptoms had spectacularly disappeared, which had often been a manifestation of their confusion and inability to commit.

Magical

Use when grounding without sinking, and protecting without shielding are called for. Like a warm blanket or a mother's soothing words, Oats bring a feeling of wellbeing and peace when exhausted, drained, or recovering from shock or upset.

Ritual

Wild oats make a lovely flower bath before rituals and celebrations, to soothe and restore. Add other flowers such as Rose, Violet, Orange Blossom, or Honeysuckle, as required.

Use at rituals for Lammas; these small seeds of potential build strength now for future challenges. Use for young men's puberty or coming-of-age rituals, to make peace with their vulnerable nature, challenging bogus masculinity, calming terror, valuing and cherishing their sensitivity but grounding it in the physical world.

White Horehound *(Marrubium vulgare)*

Mercury.
Hot 2 dry 3

Part used: herb.

Humour: melancholic.

Culpeper virtues: heats lungs, liver and spleen, cutting, opening, cleansing, discutient (scattering or dispersing).

Modern virtues: hypotensive, pectoral, anti-tussive, expectorant, antibacterial, bitter, anti-inflammatory, hypotensive, diaphoretic, antispasmodic, emmenagogue.

History

Gerard writes that Horehound syrup "is a most singular remedy against the cough and the wheezing of the lungs". He recommends it for opening the liver and spleen, cleansing the breast and lungs, and notes that it "prevails greatly against an old cough" (Woodward, 1636, p. 695). Culpeper adds, "A decoction of the dried herb and seeds or of the fresh herb taken with honey for consumptions and thin rheum on the lungs, it helps to expectorate tough phlegm from the chest with iris or oris root. It brings down the menstrua and expels the afterbirth and give ease in long labour. It expels poison. Use the leaves for foul ulcers and creeping or running sores" (Culpeper, 1798, p. 207). Culpeper quotes Galen, who said, "it cured obstructions of both the liver and the spleen and purges the lungs of phlegm, both internally and used as a poultice" (Culpeper, 1798, p. 207). Culpeper wrote that obstructions of the liver are eased by using gently binding and cleansing herbs such as Horehound, Milk Thistle, and Agrimony. As a discutient remedy, Horehound scatters the humours, and as a cleansing remedy, it carries these humours from the body. A syrup of White Horehound is used to evacuate tough phlegm and cold rheum from the lungs of aged persons, especially those who are asthmatic. Dioscorides recommends it for asthma and tuberculosis, and for "women to drive out menstrual flow and the afterbirth, for women in hard labour" (Gunther, 1968, p. 503).

Modern virtues

Horehound is known mainly as a powerful and effective cough remedy to expel and dilute thick phlegm. As an anti-tussive remedy it relieves dry, irritating, non-productive coughs. It is anti-spasmodic and so is helpful in painful periods. Its action as an emmenagogue helps with pelvic congestion and pain. As a bitter remedy it works on the liver to stimulate the production of bile, and so is helpful in digestive weakness. Its action on the liver and reproductive system is also helpful in premenstrual discomfort. As an anti-spasmodic it has been used to reduce high blood pressure caused by tension and stress.

Horehound cough drops

Make a strong infusion of the dried herb using one part strained infusion to two parts sugar.

Put in a large saucepan and boil until it reaches boiling point. To test it has candied, drop a small amount in a glass of cold water: if it forms a ball it is done. Remove from the heat and pour into a baking tray lined with parchment paper, or into a metal sweet tray. Cut into pieces when cool.

Emotional

Horehound is a plant of the upper air; it is as light and airy as a spring breeze, which has the hint of warmth to come with still the memory of winter's chill. It supports you gently and lifts you up from heavy, dull, sticky energy. It gives a cleansing by Air, which brightens lightly, uplifting, smoothing and soothing, giving a sense of calm and wellbeing. Like tai chi, it gives the illusion of lightness, but is strong and flexible, serene and flowing. Horehound offers calm serenity. It balances the energy. It gives mental clarity and is peaceful, detached, and cool.

Magical

Horehound's airy qualities are helpful when you need some perspective on a problem. Drink the tea and sit with your herb in your left hand, light a white or blue candle, and allow your mind to soar above you, like a floating cloud, high up to the upper air, and hover there like a big bird of prey. Feel the air around you as you surf the warm air currents. Slowly, turn your gaze and dispassionately look down at the issue, the people involved, and, from a place of calm, loving detachment, look at it from all angles and see what is happening and what needs to happen. Lovingly affirm that you will take the next step to resolve the issue.

Ritual

Horehound is great for group meditations. Use as a tea or an incense or a smudge, to cleanse and lighten the energy. It is especially helpful when the Moon is in Gemini or Aquarius, to escape from mundane reality. Drumming and dancing move the energy on. Use in rituals working with Air spirits and in weather work. It stimulates creativity, so use it for inspiration.

The Moon ☽

Rulerships

The Moon rules Cancer only, and is in detriment in Capricorn, exalted in Taurus, and in fall in Scorpio. She is feminine, cold and moist, and phlegmatic.

Nature

The Moon, the most familiar of the planets, waxes and wanes and travels through all twelve signs of the zodiac in around twenty-eight days. The action of the Moon is well-documented on the tides, on growth, on post-operative bleeding, on mental illness (Watson, 1971). The Moon rules the breasts, the menstrual cycle, conception, childbirth, children's illnesses, lactation, the stomach, digestion, the left eye of men, and the right eye of women.

Physically

Being cold and moist, a strong Moon or Cancer rising gives a round, soft, body and face, and a calm, welcoming appearance, which is often very attractive; the watery signs (Cancer and Pisces especially) give the most beautiful faces and bodies. They move slowly and with reticence and timidity.

Well dignified

A strong Moon will be dignified, soft, attractive, gentle, kind, sympathetic, shy and warm-hearted. They are home-bodies and domestic, motherly and caring, nurturing and honest. As Lilly observes: "one of composed manners, a soft and tender creature a lover of all honest and ingeneous sciences, a searcher and delighter of novelties" (Lilly, 1647, p. 81). The Moon is changeable; lunar types wax and wane with their moods. They avoid discord and ugliness but can be contentious with their passive aggression.

Poorly dignified

The Moon gives a lazy, escapist mindset, which may be expressed through addictions, especially to alcohol. They are lacking in drive and initiative, content with little, having low or no ambition. They may be parasitical and rely on others to support them. A tendency towards lack of movement and over-eating can cause obesity in lunar types. They are passive, negative and fearful, indecisive, self-obsessed, and over-sensitive, often lacking a sense of identity. Lilly adds, with his usual vigour: "unsteadfast, wholly caring for the present times, timorous, prodigal and easily frightened ... A meer vagabond, idle person, hating labour, a drunkard, a sot, one of no spirit or forecast, delighting to live beggarly and carelessly" (Lilly, 1647, p. 81).

Illnesses

The Moon shows menstrual problems, infertility, issues with lactation, dysmenorrhoea, heavy periods, gut ache, diseases in the left side of the body, watery discharges, diarrhoea, leucorrhoea, phlegm, catarrh, wet coughs, any disease of cold, and symptoms of heavy, dull, unremitting pain. The Moon gives conditions of unconsciousness (for it rules the brain), such as epilepsy, fainting, dementia, and brain-fog. The Moon's low energy shows exhaustion, and post-viral conditions of weakness with depression and lassitude. In babies, the Moon can indicate colic. Anxiety, fears, nightmares, hauntings, and terror are ruled by the Moon. Culpeper writes; "Under the Moon is the Bulk of the brain, the stomack, the bowels, the bladder, the taste, the left eye of a man, the right eye of a woman" (Culpeper, 1651a, p. 99). Lilly gives the Moon to "surfeits, rotten coughs convulsion fits, the falling sickness, small pox and the measles" (Lilly, 1647, p. 82).

Herbs

Cold, numbing herbs are under the Moon: Lettuce, Cabbage, Melon, Poppy, Mandrake, Willow, Cucumber, Henbane, Cleavers, Chickweed.

Miscellaneous

The Moon rules Monday and the first and eighth hours after sunrise. Her enemy is Saturn and Mars. With the Sun she forms the "lights" in a chart, showing nature. She will also show the mother. She is happy in the third and seventh house of the horoscope. The Moon signifies how a person experienced their childhood, which may be germane to any presenting conditions. She rules winter and old age—although some people give her to babyhood. I would argue both, as there are similarities between infancy and extreme old age, in my opinion.

"The Moon is a planet mean between good and bad, moderately cold and moist … it is the generator of humidity by which the whole universe is moistened … and is the fountain of peculiar influences" (Culpeper, 1798, p. 16).

General characteristics

Appearance: the Moon shows juicy, thick-leaved plants, waterish or growing by water, sweet-tasting, fast-growing in damp places.
Element: water.
Qualities: cold and moist.
Temperament: phlegmatic.
Function: expulsion.
Organs: breast, stomach and brain.
Realm: animal virtue, the brain.
Sense: sight with the Sun.
Herbs in this book: Lettuce, Mouse-Ear, Speedwell, White Willow Bark.
Herbs in *A Woman's Book of Herbs* (Brooke, 2018): Chickweed and Cleavers.
Under Culpeper: Cabbage, Adder's Tongue, Colewort, Columbines, Watercress, Moonwort, Mouse Ear, Poppies, Purslane, White Rose, White Saxifrage, Willow.

Lettuce *(Lactuca virosa)*

Moon.
Parts used: herb and root.
Cold 2 moist 2 (Gerard gives cold in 3 or 4).
Chakra: the heart.
Culpeper virtues: hypnotic, cooling, avoid in respiratory disease, cooling remedy for whole body.
Modern virtues: narcotic, sedative, anodyne, nervine, febrifuge, bitter.

History

Gerard says Lettuce "cooleth the heat of the stomacke, heartburning", it helps Choler and quenches thirst and brings on sleep, "it hindereth the generation of seed and venerous imaginations" (Woodward, 1636, p. 310). Dioscorides agrees, "the seed turns away lustful dreams" (Gunther, 1968, p. 291). Culpeper recommends the juice mixed with oil of Rose, applied to the forehead to procure sleep or easing headache from a hot cause (such as excess exercise, alcohol, coffee, anger, hot climate, sunstroke, etc.), and also for griping pains in the stomach due to Choler. It tempers the heat of the urine, the liver, and kidneys. He cautions not to use it in breathlessness or lung problems or with people who spit blood (possibly tuberculosis). He uses it for excess Choler in the heart, shown by a swift, full pulse, and anger or restlessness. It is cooling and good for a dry stomach, as shown by thirst, an appetite for dry food, and a tendency to constipation (Culpeper, 1798, p. 222). Lettuce is one of the lesser cold seeds,[14] which are useful to cool inflammation and infections, such as cystitis. Culpeper recommends Lettuce for heart conditions brought about by heat and dryness and anger, together with Borage, Purslane and Sorrel (Tobyn, 1997, p. 204).

Modern virtues

Lettuce is an effective painkiller in the treatment of migraine, stress headache, menstrual cramps or hot inflammation in the joints or anywhere in the body. It has an action similar to opium but without the side effects or addictive action. Lettuce is useful in insomnia mixed with

---

[14]The others are Succory, Endive and Purslane (Tobyn, 1997, p. 211).

Lavender, Limeflower or Hops as a tea or tincture. It is a useful remedy in hot, irritating dry coughs, to bring up stuck phlegm and lubricating, soothing, and relaxing the bronchial tubes in whooping cough and asthma. Another great remedy for anxiety and hyperactivity, Lettuce's cold nature cools down and calms a hyperactive or super-reactive nervous system, to give breathing space and calm. To recover from surgery and trauma, for the soft sleep of death, the grave and the death bed, it provides a gentle drifting off.

Emotional

Heavy, solid, sinking, Lettuce is for deep rest, physically, emotionally and mentally. To recover, re-balance, re-orientate. It is slow, slow, slow, and brings a warm, velvety darkness, an empty calm, giving the psyche time and space to heal, for respite from emotional trauma. Lettuce cools the brain from feverish thoughts, overthinking, intrusive thoughts, fears and phobias. It brings the energy down from the brain to the heart where it can be processed with love and compassion, and raises up fears from the solar plexus to the heart, to be cleansed of lower energies. It helps to calm panic, nightmare, and distorted perceptions (all lunar in origin) and bring the deep silence of the heart. Lettuce is strong and narcotic, use with care and sparingly.

Magical

Lettuce binds fear; put a sachet under the pillow for nightmares, carry it with you for panic attacks, and hold tight until it passes. It helps to ride the waves of deep and powerful emotions, to harness their power but not be drowned by them. Lettuce connects with deep, elemental Water energy. It can be scary, but it is incredibly powerful, best for grounded people or group work. On a more mundane level, water has a connection with money, and Lettuce can be used in money spells and abundance work; burn it as incense, or carry some in your purse.

Ritual

Lettuce is especially for Moon rituals in Water signs, Pisces and Cancer. Use it for deep, journeying to the ancestors to connect with deep, ancient energies, or for rituals of crones or elders. Use in Samhain rituals, going down into the underground, dark into pre-history. Its watery nature releases the flow of blocked-up energies, to shed the past and be cleansed of old pain, sloughing off the past like a snake shedding its skin. Magically, it is like pouring blessed water through the crown chakra until the whole body and aura are covered with glowing, watery energy. Use it for the dying, and in rituals for the newly-dead to let them go, allowing them to release the physical and ascend through the light. Use it also for the panic of the dying, to help them to release with ease, connecting with their hearts and surrendering into the peace of emptiness, silence, darkness, and the grave.

Mouse-Ear *(Philosella officinalis [Hieracium pilosella])*

Ruler: the Moon.
Part used: herb.
Cool 1 moist 1.
Culpeper virtues: hepatic, anti-lithic, astringent, expectorant.
Modern virtues: digestive, diaphoretic, diuretic, tonic, astringent, cholagogue, expectorant.

History

Culpeper writes, "this is a small plant possessing great virtues". A decoction helps jaundice if taken for a long time, "it is a special remedy against the stone, and gripping pains of the bowels" (Culpeper, 1798, p. 254). Mixed with Succory and Centaury it is helpful for dropsy (oedema) and diseases of the spleen. It "stayeth the fluxes of the blood" (Culpeper, 1798, p. 254), both inward and outward. Culpeper used it with his lunar tincture, of which he says: "To stay the abundance of women's courses, and to keep them in due proportion and regular, no medicine in the whole of the *Materia Medica* was ever found so efficacious ... the inherent virtues of which contain the salubrious qualities of this and other lunar herbs congenial to the female sex" (Culpeper, 1798, p. 254).[15] Traditionally, Mouse Ear as a syrup was specific for whooping cough.

---

[15]Other lunar herbs might include Shepherd's Purse.

Modern virtues

For a dry, hacking cough, with heat and fever, Mouse-Ear combined with Mullein and White Horehound makes a helpful remedy. Being cold it helps to stop bleeding and discharges, both internally and externally. It is a useful first aid kit remedy for boils and cuts, used as a powder directly on the affected area. It is a bitter, and so is a useful liver remedy taken as a tea. Used with Shepherd's Purse and Sage for flooding at the menopause and heavy periods due to fibroids, or for heavy discharges related to coldness or over-relaxation. Recent research has suggested it might have anti-radical activity against cancer cells (Gawrońska-Grzywacz et al., 2011).

Emotional

Mouse-Ear has a light and airy nature, it is uncomplicated and joyful. It gives a dose of light and laughter to people who have lost their joy temporarily. Uncomplicated and happy, it is impossible not to smile with its beguiling energy.

Magical

Drink the tea to chase away rainy-day blues. Grow it in the garden or window box for a happy home life, or at work for easy relationships with co-workers. It is modest and straightforward. Use when life feels complicated and dreary, to re-capture the joy and pleasure of simple things.

Ritual

A lovely herb for Beltane and midsummer rituals as an incense, or add in pre-ritual baths to get into a spirit of fun and celebration. Use for handfastings and naming ceremonies.

Speedwell *(Veronica officinalis)*

Moon.
Part used: herb.
Cool 1 moist 1.
Chakra: crown, ajna.

Culpeper virtues: expectorant, pulmonary.
Modern virtues: vulnerary, blood purifier, astringent, bitter, diaphoretic, tonic, expectorant, alterative, diuretic, heart tonic.

History

Speedwell was used in Wales for bleeding from the lungs, coughs, for diseases of the skin and the kidneys, and externally for wounds.

Modern virtues

As a tea or a decoction, Speedwell is used for coughs and catarrh and is a useful addition for hot and irritating skin conditions, such as chickenpox, measles, eczema and hot rashes. Believed to regenerate the stomach lining, Speedwell is a useful addition to inflamed, hot stomach, and gut conditions. It is a blood purifier, a diuretic and diaphoretic, and is helpful for eczema when mixed with Nettle, and in an ointment or lotion with Violet and Chickweed to cool and soothe. Mixed with Plantain, it is a soothing, cooling, pulmonary remedy for hot, dry, spasmodic coughs. Its moistening, expectorant action liquifies and expels mucus. Speedwell makes a good heart tonic mixed with Violet or Rose.

Emotional

Speedwell as a tea or a flower remedy, or in drop-doses, is useful for anxiety caused by over-stimulation and mental exhaustion. It calms a feverish mind and is soothing, relaxing and cooling but not sedating. It gives a peacefulness and mental clarity and helps to banish intrusive or ruminating thoughts. Speedwell strengthens the emotional body after trauma, and helps to heal the deep, deep sadness of abuse, abandonment, and familial trauma or ancestral issues. It brings a renewed self-confidence and calmness, healing the inner child and separating from family history, by building self-esteem and a sense of security. Useful in night terrors and feelings of being haunted.

Magical

Speedwell works on the ajna or third-eye chakra and is useful in clairvoyance and deep seeing, deepening meditation while at the same time keeping the person grounded and connected. Speedwell also works on the crown chakra to open a person up to spiritual energies and to bring a higher vibration into meditation or rituals. Sprinkle on the graves of restless spirits, or in houses or places where ghosts wander. Put in the coffins or graves of people who die sudden or very traumatic deaths (such as accidents or suicides). Make a strong decoction or sprinkle in the room where someone has died to send the spirit on.

Ritual

Because the flowers are tiny, Speedwell is used for evoking subtle energies, delicate Moon magic or rituals for babies or children. It may be helpful in puberty to open up to spiritual energies, while keeping the person grounded. Use as a flower remedy or a meditation tool. Use in midwinter rituals for the returning of the light, and at Samhain to make amends to the dead and release restless spirits. Use in meditation before astral travelling or vision-questing.

White Willow Bark *(Salix alba)*

Moon.
Part used: bark.
Cold 2 dry 2/3.
Culpeper virtues: cephalic, astringent without sharpness, dries up humours, cleansing, cools head and joints, hardening, binding, cleansing, cools the heart and joints.
Modern virtues: analgesic, anti-pyretic, anti-inflammatory, cardiac.

History

Gerard writes that its green branches: "doe mightily coole the heat of the aire which thing is wonderful refreshing to the sick patient" (Woodward, 1636, p. 1392). Willow, being cold and dry, dries up secretions.[16] Culpeper writes: "the leaves, bark and seed are used to staunch bleeding at the nose and mouth ... and all other fluxes of blood from either men or women" (Culpeper, 1798, p. 386). Culpeper quotes Galen,

---

[16]Culpeper mentions five other cold and dry, hardening herbs: Rose, Horsetail, Plantain, Comfrey, Shepherd's Purse (Tobyn, 1997, p. 210).

who recommends Willow to dry up humours "without any sharpness or corrosion" (Culpeper, 1798, p. 386).

Modern virtues

The Willow is the tree from which salicylates were first extracted to make aspirin. Unlike aspirin, Willow contains tannins, which mitigate against the tendency to bleed caused by salicylates. However, it should be used with caution, or avoided as a precaution by people taking warfarin and other anti-coagulants. Use for joint pain, headache, migraine, period pain, neuralgia, fevers with bone pain, fibromyalgia, and other musculoskeletal conditions, and for dull, aching, persistent phlegmatic types of pain, such as is found in cold headache and bone pain. As a cleansing medicine, Willow expels humours from the body; heavy, waterlogged conditions will improve with Willow. It is a useful addition to sleep mixes, especially for people with nerve pain, and for the pain of chickenpox and shingles. Locally, a strong decoction is useful for bleeding and painful gums. It works well mixed with Myrrh or Thyme for their antiseptic properties. Aspirin is used as a preventative for heart attacks, and White Willow can be used in the same way.

Emotional

Willow has an incredibly light, airy, expanding nature without being fiery. It is indicated for people who are temporarily stuck or who have come off their path or lost connection with their centre. For dull, heavy emotions, which cloud a person's ability to move forwards, and who are feeling despondent and lethargic, its brightness opens out the energy. Its light, expanding energy means it is not useful for ungrounded people who need more grounding and focusing energies. For people who have experienced terrible emotional pain, after trauma, which has left them feeling ripped apart, Willow helps to dull the pain, panic, and terror, so that some peace can be achieved, and healing can begin. Willow has the quality of transcending the physical body to bring peace. Willow brings lightness and optimism if someone has intolerable burdens, or is trapped inside for some reason, such as new mothers, carers, the incarcerated, the paralysed or long-term sick. Willow is one of the Bach flower remedies, recommended for resentment, self-pity, for people feeling that life has treated them unfairly, for complainers and moaners, and for overcoming sadness and grief.

Magical

Willow creates a positive environment and blocks negativity. It is such a magical plant; its lunar energies are very strong. It has the quality of solitary journeys on water in the moonlight, both an incredible stillness and connection with the stars and heavens, and the tumble and rustle of night-time creatures. It can be used as a smudge for astral travelling, dream work, meditation, or burn it as an incense with Juniper berries and other herbs as desired. Willow is a useful herb for solitary practitioners. It has a strong protective energy and can be used in binding and blocking spells to stop people harming you. Use in business to protect against misfortune. The powerful protective energies make Willow a useful herb in maji (see p. 127) as it has implacable force.

Ritual

A lovely herb to use at the full moon, especially the watery moons of Cancer and Pisces. Its light, starry energy would be good for initiation rituals or celebratory rituals. Its solitary nature also favours the lone practitioner. Use it for clearing heavy energy, after intense work with people. It is a herb of the high priestess, and is used in rituals to celebrate this aspect of the goddess: female wisdom, a deep knowing not of this world, Isis, Athene, very ancient female wisdom. Use for Moon magic, lunar blessings, healing spells.

Choosing a remedy

Time

Each day of the week is attributed to a planet: Monday, Moon; Tuesday, Mars; Wednesday, Mercury; Thursday, Jupiter; Friday, Venus; Saturday, Saturn; Sunday, Sun.

Each hour of the day is also given to a planet. The first hour after sunrise is ruled by the same planet as rules the day, i.e. on Sunday the first hour after sunrise is ruled by the Sun, then the hour afterwards by Venus, then Mercury, the Moon, Saturn and Jupiter, and then the Sun again. The eighth and first hours, then, will be governed by the same planet. The eighth will generally be around early afternoon, which is the ideal time for harvesting herbs in any case and when their planetary energies will be the most concentrated or available in the plant.

You can also use electional astrology to find the most auspicious time to pick a particular herb, which would be most important for rare plants and if they were being used for ritual or spell work. An electional chart is a horoscope for a time you elect to do something. You chose a time, draw up the chart and see what the astrology is. Culpeper gives some guidelines:

i)   Let the planet which governs the herb be angular; that is, on the ascendant, descendant, midheaven or IC.[1]

ii) Let the Moon be in good aspect and not in the houses of her enemies, i.e. not in aspect to Mars or Saturn nor in the first, eighth, tenth or eleventh houses.

I generally pick my herbs on their planetary day the week before full moon and make my tinctures as near as possible to the full moon and leave them for a lunar month, pressing them out again as near as possible to the time of the full moon, because I feel this potentises their properties.[2] The day and planetary hour is usually recorded on the decumbiture map and will be another pointer to the illness and its cause. Paracelsus (1493–1541) rejected humoral theory, but nevertheless argued it was important to find the remedy which connected what was above with what was below: "The Physician should know how to bring about a conjunction between the astral Mars and the grown Mars (i.e. the herbal remedy). In this sense the remedy should be prepared in the star and should become a star … as a remedy cannot act without the heavens, it must be directed by them" (Goodrick-Clarke, 1999, p. 75).

Virtue

This is the *materia medica* of herbs, including their usage within the context of astrology and humoral pathology, their physical, emotional, and psychic use. It includes the complexion of the patient and is understood in terms of planetary symbolism and humoral factors. Consider in your prescription:

i)   The nature of the herbs.
ii) The properties of the herbs.
iii) The elemental qualities of the herbs.
iv) The effects of the herbs.
v)   The complexion of the patient.

---

[1] Astrological terms are explained on p. 149.
[2] Always bless and thank the plant before you pick it. The more sacred your harvesting practice, the more powerful your remedies. There is a prayer in *A Woman's Book of Herbs* (Brooke, 2018, p. 215) which can be used, or develop your own invocation or blessing.

Number

i) The essential dignity and debilities of planets.
   This refers to the essential dignities and debilities of the planets according to Ptolemy's table (Appendix 2). The numbers are added, and the planet with the greatest number of points is deemed to be the strongest. The proportions of the medicine can then be adjusted according to the strongest planet.
ii) Selecting the right herbs in the right quantities and proportions.
   I work with drop doses, so I have not experimented with this. But using larger quantities of teas and tinctures it would be possible to alter the relative strengths and weaknesses according to the essential dignities of the planets.

Sympathy and antipathy

As discussed above, to treat with sympathy is to treat with nature, it is to find the cause of the illness and then to treat *similia similibis* ("like with like"). To treat by antipathy is to treat against nature, to fight the illness rather than build up the strength of the body. Allopathic medicine is a good example of treatment by antipathy. Antibiotics are used to kill the invading organism; the sympathetical approach would be to take remedies to build up the body's immune system, which would fight the pathogens, without injuring other organisms. Treating by sympathy is the bedrock of all natural therapeutics, nourishing the soil (the human organism) so the body can fight the disease as nature intended it to do. Of course, in acute medicine antibiotics can be life-saving, but over-use and resistant strains have weakened their effects, and side effects of long-term use are well-documented. In sympathetic treatment, the organs of elimination are supported: liver, kidneys, the lymphatic system, and the body takes care of its self. Within herbalism antipathetic treatment can be used (for example for pain-killing) until the patient is stabilised and wholistic treatment is initiated.

CHOOSING A REMEDY

1. TIME: *planets *planetary hours *season *cycles of the sun and moon (acute and chronic conditions) *judicial days and critical days

2. VIRTUE: *the elemental and planetary virtues of the remedy *the complexion (Temperament) of the patient

3. NUMBER: *the essential dignities of the planets. *the quantities and proportions of the remedy

4. SYMPATHY: *treating like with like *strengthening nature

5. ANTIPATHY: *opposing the sickness: (hot for cold, moist for dry)

FROM THE DECUMBITURE: choose

1. A herb of the nature of the Lord of the Ascendant

2. A herb antipathetic to Lord of the Sixth

3. One of the nature of the sign Ascending

4. If the Lord of the Tenth is strong, use his medicines

5. Or else the medicine of the Lord of time

6. Fortify the body with Sympathetical remedies

7. Regard the Heart and sustain it.

A little bit of philosophy

We have looked at the elements, the four temperaments, astrology, and *materia medica*. Now I would like to discuss humoral philosophy.

Firstly, we shall discuss how the body is composed and how it functions. This is from the top down, or from the most subtle energies to the coarsest.

The seven natural things (after Galen)[1]

1. *Spirit*: Culpeper describes it as an airy substance which permeates the brain (via the nerves), the heart (via the arteries), and the liver (via the veins). Spirit is the energy behind their various operations. When the spirit is depleted the whole body suffers. The spirit can be likened to qi or prana.
2. *Element*: the four elements from which all natural things are made: Fire, Air, Water, and Earth. Heat and cold are active; dryness and moisture passive.

---

[1] From *Galen's Art of Physick* (Culpeper, 1652, p. 5).

155

The Seven Natural Things

Spirit

The Four Elements

The Four Temperaments

The Four Humours

The Anatomy or Structure of the Body

The Faculties of the body (the Virtues & Spirits)

The Operations of the Body

3. *Complexions (Temperaments)*: the actions of these elements on the body. When Fire predominates, they are choleric; Water, phlegmatic; Air, sanguine; Earth, melancholic.
4. *Humours*: Choler, whose receptacle is in the gallbladder; Blood, whose seat is the liver; Phlegm, placed in the lungs; Melancholy, in the spleen.

The elements, complexions and humours are subservient to each other, in the same way the spirit, soul, and body are.

5. *Members*: can be simple or compound.
   Simple: bones, cartilage, ligaments, veins, arteries, nerves, tendons, fat, flesh, and skin.
   Compound: head, heart, liver, lungs, legs, arms, hands.
   Principal: brain, heart, liver, testicles.
   Subservient: nerves to carry the animal spirit, arteries to carry the vital spirit, veins to carry the natural spirit, spermatic vessels to carry the procreative spirit.

6. *Virtues*: vital virtue, natural virtue, animal virtue (see below).
7. *Operations*: of these virtues on the body.

Animal virtue:

Imagination, apprehension, fancy, opinion, and consent in the two former ventricles of the brain.

Judgment, esteem, reason, resolution, disposing, and discerning in the middle ventricle of the brain.

Remembering and forward planning in the back ventricle of the brain.

Vital virtue:

Joy, mirth, singing, by dilating the heart.
Sadness, sorrow, fear, sighing, by compressing the heart.

Natural virtue:

Transforms food into chyle, chyle into blood and humours, blood into flesh.

Joins, forms, increases, and nourishes the body.

Culpeper describes these in more detail in *Pharmacopoeia Londinensis* (Culpeper, 1653).

There are two principal virtues in the body: conservation and procreation.

Virtue of procreation

This is found in the reproductive organs of men and women and is governed principally by Venus. This virtue is augmented and fortified by herbs of Venus, diminished and cleansed by herbs of Mars, and extinguished by herbs of Saturn.

Virtue of conservation

This is divided into three parts:

	Vital virtue	Natural virtue	Animal virtue
Found in:	Heart	Liver	Brain
Governed by:	Sun	Jupiter	Mercury, Moon
Dispersed by:	Arteries	Veins	Nerves
Provides:	Vital spirit	Nourishment	Sense and reason

Vital virtue

Or "vital spirits", residing in the heart and dispersed by the arteries. These cause mirth, joy, hope, trust, humanity, mildness, courage, and their opposites: sorrow, despair, envy, hatred, stubbornness, and revenge. Vital spirits give the body its innate and acquired energy (like qi or prana). They can be depleted by excess work, worry, drugs, alcohol, insomnia, and sexual activity. The vital spirit is strengthened by herbs of the Sun: St. John's Wort, Angelica, Rosemary, Centaury, Chamomile, Marigold.

Natural virtue

Or "natural spirits" nourish the body and give it sense and motion throughout, in the same way vital spirit quickens it (gives it energy). Residing in the liver, the natural spirits' work is to alter and concoct food and to transform it into chyle, from chyle to blood, from blood to flesh, in order to form, engender, nourish, and increase the body. The four humours come from the liver: blood, choler, phlegm, and melancholy.

Blood

Blood makes flesh, and any excess makes seed (sperm, eggs). Its receptacle is the veins, and it is dispersed by the veins throughout the body. Blood nourishes the judgement and fortifies the digestive faculty. It is ruled by Jupiter. It is the first-produced humour. Its superfluities (excess) then produce choler, the fiery superfluity; then phlegm, the watery superfluity; and finally melancholy, the earthy superfluity.

Choler

Choler clarifies (separates and cleanses) all humours, heats the body, and nourishes the apprehension. It fortifies the attractive faculty, and it moves a person to activity and valour. It is ruled by Mars and its receptacle is the gallbladder.

Phlegm

Phlegm fortifies the expulsive faculty, makes the body slippery, and allows the body to expel substances. It fortifies the brain by its similarity to it (cold and moist) and spoils apprehension by antipathy (apprehension being hot and dry). It qualifies Choler and moistens the heart, therefore sustaining it and the whole body from the fiery effects continual motion would cause. Its receptacle is the lungs and it is governed by Venus and the Moon.

Melancholy

Melancholy is the sediment of blood, cold and dry in quality. It fortifies the retentive faculty and memory, "makes men sober, solid and staid, fit for study; staies the unbridled toyes and fooleries of lustful blood, stays the wandring thoughts, and reduceth them home to the Centre: it is like a grave Counsellor to the whole Body" (Culpeper, 1651b, n.p.). Its receptacle is the spleen and it is governed by Saturn.

Animal virtue

It lives in the brain and it is ruled by Mercury and the Moon as both planets can either fortify or impede it. The Moon is the sensitive part of the brain, and Mercury the rational part. In a chart where the Moon is stronger than Mercury, senses overpower reason, and the opposite is true: if Mercury is stronger, then reason overcomes the senses. The animal virtue is divided into two parts, intellective and sensitive.

Intellective

This is governed by Mercury and is divided into imagination, judgement and memory.

Imagination

Imagination is found in the forebrain and is hot and dry. It is quick, active, and always working. It receives vapours from the heart and makes them into thoughts. It never sleeps; only when judgement is awake is it regulated. When judgement is asleep it runs at random and forms any thought according to the nature of the vapour sent up to it. Mercury disposes of it.

Judgement sleeps when men do; imagination never sleeps; and memory sometimes sleeps and sometimes not. When memory is awake and the person sleeps, this produces dreams.

Dreams are one of the best ways to see the humour or complexion predominating in the body.

- Sanguine dreams show groups of people, lots of colour, bright, hopeful, cheerful images. Scenes showing beauty, celebrations, parties, love and play, spring flowers. Overall, sanguine dreams are happy, celebratory, feel-good, and expansive. They include travel, people from other countries, opulence, and indulgence.
- Choleric dreams are, predictably, of fire and movement; flames, flying, swift and angry action, fighting, arguments, violence, climbing higher, impossible achievements, ambition, and thirst for power. Also: deserts, heat, irritability, fevers, passion, lust, and selfishness.
- Phlegmatic dreams reflect the languor of the humour: lazy dreams, crawling, fear of falling, drowning, water, the sea, nightmares and hauntings. Also: images of angels, spirits, gods and goddesses, magical beings, faeries, and other mythical creatures.
- Melancholic dreams are sad, heavy, and feature tombs, bats, owls, darkness, solitude, loneliness, fear, skulls, ghosts. They are often set at night. Also, they may show exams, tests for which the dreamer is unprepared, naked, exposed, or shamed. Also: study, books, old age, old people, seriousness.

The condition of Mercury in the natal chart will show what kind of imagination a person has. A fiery Mercury will show creativity, but perhaps no sustained effort; a watery Mercury, great depth but fearful; airy Mercury, lots of ideas but unstable or flighty; and earthy Mercury, high intelligence but conservative.

Judgement

Judgement is seated in the middle of the brain to show it ought to rule over imagination and memory, the ruler of the little (personal) world. Judgement's job is to approve of what is good and reject what is bad. It is the seat of reason and the judge of actions. All failings are committed through its infirmity, and in not judging correctly between a real and an apparent good. It is ruled by Jupiter and is hot and moist.

Memory

Situated in the back of the brain, memory is the great register to the little world. Its office is to record things either done and past or to be done. It is cold and dry and melancholic. Generally, melancholic types are the most tenacious in every way and have the best memory (or those with a strong Saturn or Mercury, on the ascendant, or mid-heaven, or conjunct the Sun or Moon). Memory is under Saturn and purged by the luminaries (Sun and Moon).

Sensitive

The second part of the animal virtue is the sensitive virtue, which is divided into two parts: common sense and particular sense.

Particular senses

The particular senses are regulated and united by common sense, but each one is independent.

Sight

Sight is cold and moist and resides in the eye. It governed by the luminaries (the Sun rules the right eye in men and the left eye in women, the Moon vice versa). People with afflicted Sun or Moon in their horoscope often have poor eyesight or suffer from eye problems.

Hearing

Hearing is cold and dry and melancholy and resides in the ears and is ruled by Saturn, although Mercury, too, can show deafness.

Smell

Smell is hot and dry, resides in the nose, is choleric, and is ruled by Mars, which is why choleric creatures such as dogs have a good sense of smell.

Taste

Taste is hot and moist and resides in the palate, and discerns whether food is good to eat or not. However, desire can override this sense, and food is eaten which is harmful, although taste does discern poisonous or rotten food well. It is ruled by Jupiter and the sanguine humour, which has a great appetite, but can harm itself by over-indulgence.

Feeling

Feeling is located all over the body and combines all the qualities, hot, cold, moist, and dry. It is the index of all tangible things: hot feels hot, and cold, cold. Feeling relates to the sensations the whole body feels (shivering with cold, sweating with heat, etc.) Culpeper gives this to Mercury.

Common Sense

Common sense unites the particular senses in harmony (or not) and is ruled by Mercury, which, as Culpeper suggests is "why men are so fickle headed" (Culpeper, 1651b, n.p.).

These are the principle virtues which control the body. I particularly like the threefold vital, natural, and animal spirits. Plato separated the soul into three parts: the intellect (νους) or mind, understanding, reason, thought, insight, purpose, intention, and meaning; the nobler affections (θυμος) or courage, spirit, passion, and anger; and the appetites (επιθυμια) or desire, longing, wishes, and lust. We might describe them (respectively) as the higher mind in the brain, or the higher centres, like the ajna and crown chakras; the heart chakra, where we experience universal love and noble emotions such as courage or righteous anger; and the liver or solar plexus chakra, where our appetites and desires are fed and experienced.

Feeding the heart, for example, cultivates the nobler emotions and helps us to rise above petty, selfish, and cruel feelings. It is well known that our emotional lives and experiences affect the physical heart; people do die of a broken heart. People who are aggressive and selfish and driven are more likely to suffer from heart conditions, as are people who cannot make meaningful (heart-based) connections with other people.

The liver, of course, is concerned with digestion and absorption of nourishment. We have a vocabulary which expresses emotional discomfort in terms of these appetites, where "we cannot stomach something", "we cannot swallow or digest an insult", or "it makes me feel sick". Appetites reside in the liver; addictions, cravings, selfishness, describe an emotional baby state where we cannot rise to the higher centres of love, but are stuck in a needy, greedy, cycle of appetite.

Herbs, of course, with help this. The easiest to demonstrate are the herbs for the heart: Rose, Melissa, Motherwort, Violet, Hawthorn, Yarrow, and Rosemary, which all, in their different ways, soothe, strengthen, and open the heart chakra. They bring awareness of love, they heal the frightened or hurt heart, and they restore faith and re-orientate the emotions in their correct location, the centre for love.

Liver remedies have a powerful effect, not only on the physical liver but on the emotional and spiritual liver. They cleanse both this magnificent organ of elimination, but also the lesser emotions, which often cause or are companions to liver complaints: anger, jealousy, resentment, bitterness, selfishness, and greed. By keeping the energy flowing through the liver these toxic emotions, which we all have at one time or another, can be diluted, neutralised, and washed away.

The brain as the seat of reason, judgement, memory and imagination fits well with the throat, brow, and crown chakras as they create, express, and channel higher and more spiritual energies. The lower, "monkey mind" is exemplified by Mercury, which, as you will remember, takes on the energy of whatever is near. The mind can be trained in meditation to be calm, serene, and full of wisdom and creative insights, or it can run wild, jabbering and chattering, filling the thoughts with fear, worry, and negativity. The higher mind needs both the wide-open spaces of Jupiter to soar, question, and explore as well as the rigor and structure of Saturn to ground in everyday practice the insights it has discovered.

Of particular interest to practitioners in locating the complexion are dreams. A simple question concerning the narrative in dreams usually indicates a temperament, while enquiry into recent dreams, occurring during the time of the sickness, will point to a temporarily acquired temperament and suggest a treatment regimen.

The administering virtue

While the principal virtues are concerned with procreation and conservation, as we have seen above, the administering virtue is concerned with how the body, mind, and spirit attracts, absorbs, retains, and expels nourishment; how it experiences and expresses emotions and spiritual energies. It can be sub-divided into the following.

Attractive virtue

This is hot and dry (so has energy and initiative) and is ruled by Mars and the Sun. Its job is to attract what the body needs physically, emotionally, and spiritually. In terms of treatment, Culpeper suggests strengthening this virtue by taking medicines or other treatments when the Moon is in a Fire sign or when the ascendant of the decumbiture (see p. 212) is a Fire sign and using herbs of the Sun and Mars.

Digestive virtue

This is the main aspect of the administering virtue, and the "others like handmaidens attend on it" (Culpeper, 1651b, n.p.). The attractive virtue draws in what this virtue should digest, serving constantly to feed and supply it. The retentive virtue holds the substance in the body for as long as the digestive virtue needs. And the expulsive virtue casts out that which is superfluous to digestion. The digestive virtue is hot and moist, for digestion needs heat to act, and moisture to mix the food. It is under the influence of Jupiter and is fortified by its plants. The digestive virtue can be best strengthened when the Moon is in Gemini, Aquarius, or the first half of Libra, or when one of these signs is on the ascendant of the decumbiture. Scheduling treatments for these times will increase their efficacy.

Retentive virtue

This is cold and dry and under the influence of Saturn. It compresses, for this is the nature of cold, and it retains, as this is the nature of dryness, nourishment. Culpeper suggests this shows why Saturnine people are often "covetous and tenacious" (Culpeper, 1651b, n.p.). To strengthen this virtue, use the herbs of Saturn when the Moon or the ascendant is in Taurus, Virgo, or Capricorn, but not when Saturn is in the first house.

Expulsive virtue

This is cold and moist, cold because it compresses the superfluities, and moist because it makes them fit for ejection from the body. It is under the Moon and Venus. To strengthen this faculty, especially when purging the humours, so they can be removed from the body, treat when the Moon is in Cancer, Scorpio, or Pisces, or in the ascendant of the decumbiture, and use herbs of the Moon and Venus.

I really like Culpeper's explanation of how the body nourishes itself and maintains a homeostatic balance between taking in, digestion, and expulsion. In practice this can clearly be seen: sometimes the stomach is too dry, and causes constipation and indigestion; sometimes the digestive system is too wet, and food passes through undigested; sometimes, when too cold, there is bloating, stagnation, vomiting; or, when too hot, heartburn and cramps.

SPIRIT [breath pneuma]

THE FOUR ELEMENTS [the physical body]

Fire (Sun/Mars) ☉♂   Earth (Mercury/Saturn) ☿♄   Air (Jupiter) ♃   Water (Moon/Venus) ☽♀

THE FOUR FACULTIES

VITAL virtue	ANIMAL virtue	NATURAL virtue	PROCREATIVE virtue
Heart & Arteries	1.Brain	Liver & Veins	Reproductive organs
Sun ☉	Moon ☽-Sensitive	Jupiter ♃	Venus ♀
	*Taste (Jupiter) ♃		
	*Hearing (Saturn) ♄		
	*Smell (Mars) ♂		
	*Sight (Sun & Moon) ☉☽		
	*Feeling (Venus) ♀		
	*Common Sense (Mercury) ☿		
	2. Nerves		
	*Judgement (Jupiter) ♃		
	*Mercury-Intellective ☿		
	*Memory (Saturn) ♄		
	*Imagination (Mercury) ☿		

THE FOUR OPERATIONS

(Administering virtues)

*Attraction: Mars & Sun hot & dry

*Digestion: Jupiter hot & moist

*Retention: Saturn cold & dry

*Expulsion: Moon & Venus cold & wet

FOUR FLUIDS

*Blood (Jupiter) ♃

*Choler (Mars) ♂

*Phlegm (Moon & Venus) ☽♀

*Melancholy (Saturn) ♄

FOUR ORGANS

*Liver (Jupiter) ♃

*Lungs (Moon & Venus) ☽♀

*Gall Bladder (Mars) ♂

*Spleen (Saturn) ♄

Astrological medicine: background and history

Beyond the temperaments, there is a deeper method which combines two of the ancient arts, astrology and healing. Star lore was always associated with medicine. Early physicians could see the effect of lunar cycles and eclipses on nature and the body. Our earliest written reference to Greek astrology is Hesiod's *Works and Days* written in approximately 750 BCE. Hesiod, who was a farmer in Boetia, counselled that "when Orion and Sirius shall have reached mid-heaven and Arcturus shall rise with the dawn, then, O Perses, gather your grapes and bring them home" (Tester, 1987, p. 82).

Works and Days lists sixteen of the days of the month on which certain activities were unfavourable, while the fifteenth was a bad day (Tester, 1987, p. 82). Possibly Hesiod was referring to the new moon, if he was counting from the full moon, which is traditionally a bad day in horary astrology.

Medicine as an empirical science was the creation of the ancient Greeks and they linked it with astrology. Early astrology was Greek, influenced by Babylonian star lore, and was practiced in the same places where medicine was developed: Cos, Pergamum, and Alexandria, which were centres of learning and sites of large library complexes. Greeks were obsessed with classifying and ordering their world.

167

They used what they knew of the heavens to fit their own theories of how the world operated in nature and health and disease. Hippocrates and early Greek doctors understood that the environment, the seasons, phases of the moon, and climactic conditions could aggravate or improve medical conditions.

Berosus was a Babylonian priest who settled on Cos (the likely birthplace of Hippocrates) in the early fourth century BCE and is believed to have established a school of astrology there (Barton, 1994, p. 23). This shows the probability that there were connections between medicine and astrology from the beginning of Greek science. Cos had a small shrine to the Sun god and Hermera, goddess of the day, unique in the Greek world, which did not worship the Sun and Moon. The philosopher Plato (c. 428-328 BCE) was critical of the old Olympian gods, and argued it was the heavenly bodies that were divine and should be worshipped for the mathematical beauty of their movements. It is unclear if Plato was influenced by Pythagoras (569-c. 475 BCE) or Berosus or both thinkers (Tester, 1987, p. 16).

Later astrological medicine, *iatromathematica* (*iatros*, "doctor"; *mathematica*, "astronomy": ιατρομαθεματικα), was developed and rationalised by the Hellenistic Greeks living in Alexandria (Tester, 1987, p. 19). They associated plants with the heavenly bodies and signs of the zodiac. Galen used astrology, although he separated himself from "augers and astrologers" (Nutton, 2013, p. 272) claiming that his prognoses came from rational calculation and observation. However, he admitted he consulted the heavens, like Hippocrates had, using astrology as an aid to understand changes in the weather and the aetiology of disease (Nutton, 2013, p. 273). Galen mentioned the astrologer Ptolemy favourably, writing that astrology, like medicine, was a "conjectural art" and giving supreme merit to the Egyptian (Alexandrian) astrologers who united both arts (Toomer, 1985, p. 199). It is clear in Galen's *Critical Days* (Book III) that he was well-acquainted with astrology and expected his readers to be so also. Galen allowed that many of the observations of Alexandrian astrologers were true, especially with regard to the Moon and malign planets at birth.

For the Greeks, order was beautiful. The derivation of the Greek word "cosmos" (κοσμος) gives us our word "cosmetics", or beautifying aids. Greeks believed all things were one and governed by logos, the same natural law, or cosmic force and reason (λογος), and that each part affects the whole and is affected by it. Ptolemy (100–170 CE) gave an account (logos) of astronomy and astrology from the perspective of contemporary philosophical ideas. These centred around Stoicism, which promoted a philosophy of self-sufficiency and a life lived in harmony with nature. Stoics believed that although humans had free will, if they chose to live in harmony with universal spiritual laws and live with their fate (as determined by the stars) then peace could be achieved. Living contrary to these laws, and disregarding one's *daimon* ("good angel") produced a life of disappointment and pain and grief (Tester, 1987, pp. 60, 68).

In the same way that Galen missed or disregarded Dioscorides' views on *materia medica*, Ptolemy neglected the divinatory, spiritual form of astrology, *katarche* (καταρχη) and instead developed the machine of destiny model in his famous work *Tetrabiblios* (Cornelius, 1994, p. 111).

Medicine, until the eighteenth century, was Galenic, and the astrology practised in Europe comes from Ptolemy. In the same way that Galen "systematised" medical practice and gathered up all the extant medicinal knowledge of his time, which became the canon of medicine for the next 1300 years, Ptolemy rationalised and organised astrology according to his theory, which has remained unchallenged and forms the basis of Western astrology.

Both men wrote in the tradition of Greek rationalism, that is, the cosmos is so well-arranged that no part of it is independent of other parts, or of the whole (Sarton, 1959, p. 165). Astrology appealed to educated Greeks precisely because they were rational, and because astrology provided a rational system, or could be made to look like one. The Greeks mapped the heavens and then tried to interpret that map in terms of cosmic sympathy (της κοσμικης συμπαθεις) for the Greeks believed nothing happened to man which was not in sympathy with cosmic law (Tester, 1987, p. 18).

Ptolemy reflects the orthodox Greek classical position of celestial causation (cosmic sympathy). It is a mechanistic view of the world, or scientific rationalism (Cornelius, 1994, p. 87). At the centre of Ptolemy's thesis is time, the seed time when an event occurred. Ptolemy saw two effects of the planets on life: the universal and the particular. Suffused throughout the heavens and nature is the ether, which changes in the elements via the Sun and other planets, and causes the seasons and cycles. Through the circulation of ether all living things are affected. Thus, the universal or general effects of the planets affect whole countries and races with events such as famine, heatwaves, war, and pestilence.

These general effects (unlike those that are particular) cannot be timed, but are usually the result of comets and large planetary conjunctions, such as the Jupiter-Saturn conjunction at the time of the birth of Christ.

The particular effect comes into being at the moment of conception. Ptolemy contended that the planets moulded and formed the seed at that moment, and its character was fixed to such an extent that the general effect of the planets is entirely mediated by the particular. Thus, one person's experience of the general effects, say a pestilence or heatwave, would entirely depend on their particular character formed at the moment of conception.

Thus, the moment of conception is the moment of astrology for Ptolemy, which Cornelius defines as the "doctrine of origin" and the "hypothesis of seeds" (Cornelius, 1994, p. 91). Within Aristotelian logic, Ptolemy claims a "continuous process of celestial influence playing at all instants upon terrestrial affairs" (Robbins, 1940, p. 315) and offers both a rational and causal justification for events on Earth, albeit within the confines of astrological theory. This paradigm forms the basis of Western natal astrological theory.

Decumbiture

Decumbiture is a branch of horary astrology that concerns the asking of questions. A decumbiture question is about health and sickness: Will I get well? What is my illness? Which treatment will be best for me? Horary and decumbiture are *katarche* or divination, older forms of astrology than the Ptolemaic system of natal horoscopy. The moment of a horary question cannot be either a general moment nor a particular moment (Cornelius, 1994, p. 116) but "the moment of a horary is a function of human decision" (Cornelius, 1994, p. 345). This was the explanation of the twelfth-century astrologer Guido Bonatus, who translated Arabic astrology.

When a patient consults a herbalist or an astrologer there are three pivotal moments. First, there is the intention to enquire; second, the imprint of the planets on the thing asked; and, third, the free will of the questioner who then independently choses that moment to ask the question (Cornelius, 1994, p. 116). This is the *katarche* moment (or the moment of beginnings) when the patient brings their condition to the healer. Bonatus describes how the moment only exists when the question is posed and, furthermore, "whether or not the whole exercise is finally going to work is the function of an intangible, the state of the astrologer" (Cornelius, 1994, p. 345). For Bonatus, astrology is not about "objective facts" as Ptolemy suggests, but symbols which guide the participants to "fruitful action" (Cornelius, 1994, p. 345).

Therefore, *katarche*, the older, pre-rational astrology, was divination and augury, asking not what is written, but whether the action contemplated is supported by the gods. *Katarche* presupposes human participation, for the moment of divination is only significant if the question is asked. Ptolemy, with his "doctrine of the seed", brought Greek science to what had previously been ritual and divination and, in effect, replaced the gods with the machine of destiny. Ptolemy developed a perpetual ephemeris (tables of the motions of the planets) which meant that "destiny was determined by the heavens in orderly, periodic and in principle, calculable cycles" (Cornelius, 1994, p. 182). If it was written in the stars, supplication and ritual were redundant. The machine of destiny brings the fatalism of predestination. Cornelius suggests this philosophy was related to the rise of Christianity, which saw the previous, Pagan, intimate relationship with the divine as superstition and forbade it (Cornelius, 1994, p. 183). A more cynical interpretation might be that Christianity wished its adherents to lose their personal, active relationship with the divine and subscribe to a creed that intercepted, interpreted, and controlled messages from the gods to suit the purposes of the church rather than those of its members.

There is a parallel here with medicine. If the divine can only be mediated or interpreted via priests, then medicine can only be mediated by doctors. The individual cannot contact the divine, and the patient cannot be involved in their own healing. Both encourage an ethos of passivity and dependence on the expert, and a disempowering of the unqualified. We see how this doctrine had worked out by the seventeenth century in Culpeper's struggle to return healing into the hands of the ordinary people, a struggle that continues to this day.[1]

In our age, religion's power over hearts and minds has diminished and been replaced by science or *scientism*, which can be defined as: "the

---

[1]An interesting article in the *New York Times* (Joseph, 2018) related how an eminent physician, Dr. Bernard Lown, rebelled at the lack of control or even input into his treatment he was permitted while in hospital: "I always was the last to know what exactly was going on, and my opinion hardly mattered". He described how he was seen as a composite of disparate parts, which were acted upon by scientists who had lost sight of the art of healing, and lacked both common sense and empathy for his condition. "[H]ealing is replaced with treating, caring is supplanted by managing, and the art of listening is taken over by technological procedures". Dr. Lown said, "doctors of conscience" have to "resist the industrialization of their profession".

inappropriate extension of scientific method to phenomena and domains of experience which cannot be reduced to objective and positive assertions of a literal nature" (Patrick Curry, cited in Cornelius, 1994, p. 197).

Scientism claims there is only one class of truth, and that any individual experience is only valid if it fits in with this class of truth. Science has been made a substitute for philosophy in Western medicine. Herbal medicine can be analysed scientifically, the parts or active constituents can be extracted and separated out and the action on the physical body demonstrated. Western herbal medicine, like Western astrology, has fallen into the trap of scientism. Some herbalists are over-eager to cosy up to the scientific establishment, happily substituting White Willow bark for aspirin. (Salicylates were extracted from White Willow bark to make aspirin.) All well and good; arguably, White Willow bark is safer than aspirin and has the benefit of not being produced by big pharma. However, it diminishes the beauty and complexity of herbal remedies to nuts and bolts and renders the patient "done to" by the herbalist. It is my contention that, like *katarche* in astrology, herbal medicine has lost the involvement of the practitioner in the consultation, and has been diminished as a result.[2] Using the decumbiture method within the herbal practice invokes the spirit of *katarche* and brings the herbalist centre stage in the healing journey.

In continuing to locate astrology at the heart of medicine, some more history. Roman Emperor Justinian closed all the pagan philosophical schools in 529 CE. The Greeks moved east to the Persian court, taking all the scientific and medical works from the Hellenistic scholars and most of Aristotle's works. Again, like Galen, Ptolemy's writings were kept and copied into Arabic by Byzantine and Arab scholars, to remerge in Europe in the late Middle Ages when they were translated from Arabic and Greek into Latin and eventually into the vernacular languages and widely disseminated.

Both Ptolemy and Galen were part of the curriculum at the new universities of Padua, Salerno, Paris and, later, Oxford and Cambridge. Our understanding of medical astrology comes from two seventeenth-century astrologers, William Lilly and Nicholas Culpeper (see p. 189 and p. 188).

---

[2]Of course, experienced practitioners know this to be true. Within all healing, it is the relationship between the client and practitioner which is paramount, whatever the healing modality.

The men were friends and working during the time of the English Revolution, supporting the parliamentary side against the forces of the King Charles I. Because of the social and political turmoil, many of the oppressive offices of the State were closed down. This allowed them to publish works on astrology and medicine, and, in Culpeper's case, to translate the *Pharmacopoeia Londinensis* (the book of recipes of the College of Physicians) from Latin to English (Culpeper, 1653). His move was both radical—giving untrained people access to medical knowledge—and revolutionary, undermining the status quo of the university-educated medical profession.

Culpeper's work is accessible and easy to follow. He writes with a sound knowledge of his subject, and in all his books he places astrology firmly in the centre of his practice. Lilly also explores many of the rules and methods of medical astrology in his seminal work, *Christian Astrology* (1647).[3] Much of the detailed information we have on medical astrology comes from Culpeper's *Semeiotica Uranica* or *The Astrological Judgement of Diseases* (Culpeper, 1651a).

[3]See, especially, Lilly, 1647, pp. 243–296 and pp. 576–585.

Dramatis personae

This section will look at some of the people mentioned previously and how they fit in with one another and the history of astrology and medicine.

Hippocrates (c. 460-370 BCE)

Little is known of the life of Hippocrates, or even if he was born in Cos. Plato wrote about him in *Protagoras* claiming, in 430 BCE, that Hippocrates was a renowned physician and a member of the medical family that claimed descent from Asclepius, the god of healing.

The Hippocratic Corpus contains sixty works written in Ionic Greek, printed in 1526 and believed to be a compilation of the theory and practice of medicine of the third century BCE (Nutton, 2013, p. 71). Not all the books under Hippocrates' name were written by the same author, but it is agreed they were mostly written between 420-350 BCE, which may have corresponded to the lifetime of Hippocrates (Nutton, 2013, pp. 60–61). It is believed the collection was assembled in Alexandria at the famous library, when Cos was part of the Ptolomeic Empire.

The Hippocratic Corpus covers all aspects of physical and mental health. Pythagorean philosophers credited Hippocrates with aligning medicine with philosophy, teaching that disease was not punishment of the gods but due to internal and external factors such as climate and diet. It is unlikely that Hippocrates was responsible for, or believed in, the theory of the four humours. This has been attributed to his son-in-law. Hippocrates' therapeutic focus was on the healing power of nature, or *vis medicatrix naturae*, which healed the patient by supporting and strengthening his vital spirit, using rest and gentle remedies.

Although it is doubtful the Hippocratic Oath was written by Hippocrates, it remained an important part of the Hippocratic Corpus, giving rules for the ethical practice of medicine. Hippocrates was a pivotal figure in the early Hellenistic period by establishing medical theories which others could agree with or dispute (Nutton, 2013, p. 222).

Hippocrates: teachings

> [... T]he study of medicine is like the growing of plants. Our natural talent is the soil. The wisdom of our teachers is the seed. As the seed grows as does our learning, sometimes falling on fertile ground. Nourishment for our studies comes from the surrounding environment and supports its growth. Persistence in our studies is like the fertilized soil. The passage of time and experience strengthens all these things so that their nature is perfected. (Hippocrates, 1979a, p. 265, my translation.)

> So, the body of man contains Blood and Phlegm, Choler [yellow bile] and Melancholy [black bile] and these constitute his nature [temperament], because of them he suffers pain or has good health ... Pain is felt when one of these elements is deficient or in excess, or is isolated within the body, separated from the other elements. (Hippocrates, 1979b, p. 11, my translation.)

> In every illness, a positive attitude and healthy appetite is a good sign, the reverse a bad sign. (Hippocrates, 1975a, p. 103, my translation)

> With all movement of the body, when it begins to cause pain, rest at once. (Hippocrates, 1975a, p. 109, my translation.)

> Excess is hostile to nature, when changing from one regimen to another, proceed slowly. (Hippocrates, 1975a, p. 110, my translation.)

> In extreme illness, extreme remedies are precisely the most efficacious. (Hippocrates, 1975a, p. 90, my translation.)

In winter, eat warm and dry food as much as possible and drink as little as possible. In spring, drink more water and eat more vegetables. In summer, eat many vegetables both raw and cooked and cereals and diluted wine, foods which both cool and moisten the body. In autumn, decrease liquids and eat more cereals as they are drying to the body. (Hippocrates, 1975b, p. 45, my translation.)

Diseases caused by over eating are cured by fasting [and purging] those caused by purging [and fasting] are cured by feeding. (Hippocrates, 1979b, p. 25, my translation.)

[T]he contribution of astronomy to medicine is not a small one, but a very great one indeed. (Hippocrates, 1868, n.p., my translation.)

Life is short, but the art [of medicine] is long, opportunity is elusive and experience deceptive. Judgement is difficult. The physician must do what he can, the patient and their attendants should co-operate while circumstances remain favourable. (Hippocrates, 1975a, p. 98, my translation.)

Dioscorides (c. 40–80 CE)

Pedanius Dioscorides was born in Anazarbus in Turkey in the Greek-speaking eastern Roman Empire. He probably studied medicine in nearby Tarsus, which was a centre for pharmacy and pharmacology (Riddle, 1985, p. 2). He was a physician, pharmacologist, possibly an army doctor or soldier, botanist, and author of *De Materia Medica*, a five-volume pharmacology that was widely read for the next 1,500 years. Dioscorides' pharmacopoeia was the precursor for all subsequent pharmacologies, including those of Galen. It was always in circulation and was widely used until the nineteenth century in both Western and Arabic medicine. Commentaries on his text by Arab and Indian scholars helped to identify some of the more obscure plants Dioscorides discussed.

The *Materia Medica* lists the medicinal properties of about 1,000 natural products, mostly from the plant kingdom. The scale of Dioscorides' work ensured its survival. In contrast, the Hippocratic Corpus, the largest medical work surviving, lists only 130 medicines. The scale of *Materia Medica* and the fact that Dioscorides did not write about the medical theories which were being argued over at that time, meant he was not associated with one or another school of thought that subsequently fell into disuse. This ensured the survival of his *Materia Medica*, unlike other medical texts, which have been lost. Dioscorides wrote the first database of ancient pharmacy and he established the frame, form, and context for subsequent writers on *materia medica* (Riddle, 1985, p. xviii). The *Dioscorea* genus of plants was named after him by Linnaeus.

Dioscorides was the first writer to organise his pharmacopoeia by class of remedy: trees, aromatics, pot herbs, etc., and then to group his remedies to gether by their physiological actions. Previous writers simply arranged herbs alphabetically. Dioscorides, through direct observation of physical effects on the body and with the greatest of precision, classified his remedies. Botanists and doctors were baffled for centuries over his classification; it was not until the development of chemistry in the eighteenth century, pharmacognosy in the nineteenth century, and phytochemistry in the twentieth century that the logic of his system was understood. Dioscorides suggested that groupings according to physiological effects would make it easier to remember medical information. However, by not explaining his method Dioscorides' subtle and complex system was discarded by later writers, including Galen, in favour of the alphabetical pharmacopoeia (Riddle, 1985, p. 23).

Dioscorides classified most of his remedies according to: name and synonyms, habitat, botanical description, properties and actions, medicinal uses, side effects, quantities and dosages, harvesting, preparation and storage, adulteration methods and methods of testing, veterinary uses, magical and non-medical uses, specific geographical locations and habitats. The geographical location of plants affected their medicinal properties: those in mountainous, high, windswept cold and dry places yielded a stronger medicine than those collected in flat, wet places or shady places, while those collected out of season produced the weakest effect. This has been demonstrated by modern pharmacology and chemistry (Riddle, 1985, p. 29).

A good example of Dioscorides' taxonomy are the remedies containing tropane and related alkaloids: hyoscyamine, atropine, scopolamine. Dioscorides grouped them together because they have similar physiological effects, although these herbs have a different physical appearance and would not necessarily appear to be related. In the eighteenth century these herbs were classified as the Solanaceae family by Linnaeus.

It is suggested that had Dioscorides' system not be overridden by Galen, chemistry would have developed much faster in Europe, as the action of each remedy lay in the remedy itself, as Paracelsus was later to argue (Riddle, 1985, p. 175).

Dioscorides on Lettuce

The Greek word for lettuce, θριδαξ comes from τρισδακνω ("triple sting" or "hurt") referring to its bitter taste and poisonous nature. In Latin, Wild Lettuce is *lactuca virosa, lactuca* referring to its milky juice while *virosa* means poisonous (Riddle, 1985, p. 28).

> Cultivated lettuce is good for the upper tract, a little cooling, sleep causing, softening to the lower tract, increasing lactation. Boiled down it increases nutrition. Unwashed and eaten it is good for upper digestive problems. Its seeds being drunk are good for those who continually dream, and they avert sexual intercourse. Eaten too often they cause dim-sightedness. They are preserved in brine. The stalk growing up has something like the potency of the juice and sap of the wild lettuce. Wild lettuce, is similar to the cultivated, it has a larger stalk, the leaves are whiter and thinner, more rough and bitter to taste. To some degree its properties are similar to the opium poppy, thus some people mix its juice with opium. The sap in sour wine purges away watery humors through the digestive tract; it cleans away albugo (white film on the cornea) and misty eyes. It assists against the burning of the eyes anointed on with breast milk. Generally, it is sleep inducing and anodyne. It expels the menses and is given as a drink for insect bites. The seeds are given to avert dreams and sexual intercourse. Its juice produces the same things but with weaker force. (Gunther, 1968, p. 176)

Lettuce contains lactucarium, which consists of lactucin, hyoscyamine, and mannite. Hyoscyamine, present in greatest concentration in the seeds, is a tropane alkaloid and a resolution of atropine, which has a side effect of blurred vision (Dioscorides said it dulls the sight). In 1899, lactucin was discovered as an opium substitute, or rather, re-discovered 1,700 years later. Dioscorides writes that opium has a cooling property, as did all poisons, explaining the physiological effect of hyoscyamine, which is similar to opium (Riddle, 1985, p. 38).

Ptolemy (c. 100–170 CE)

Of predicting the future with astrology, Oh Syrus, two of the greatest and most powerful ways are: firstly, ordered and practically by
which we discover the configurations of the movements of the Sun,
Moon and stars, both towards one another, and in relation to the
earth. Secondly, through the effects the natural qualities of these
configurations have on the environment. The first, has its own
theory and method explained in my book the *Almageist*. The second,
less self-sufficient, shall be explained in this book [*The Tetrabiblos*]
through philosophy. (Robbins, 1940, p. 3, my translation.)

Claudius Ptolemy was a philosopher, mathematician, astronomer,
astrologer, and geographer, believed to have been born and to have
lived in Alexandria, which was the scientific and cultural capital of
the age. Alexandria had a cosmopolitan population; scholars, philosophers, doctors, and scientists flocked to study at the famous library and
Museum (the temple of the muses, goddesses of the arts). The Museum
was a research institute, and scholars were supported by the State.
It is said that each ship which docked at the port of Alexandria had to
submit any learned text to the library, to be copied and added to the collection. Galen and Dioscorides studied medicine there.

Ptolemy gave an account (*logos*) of both astronomy (*astro*, "star";
nomia, "law") and astrology (*astro*, "star"; *logos*, "discourse") which was
scientific and in sympathy with the philosophy of the time. Like Galen
with medicine, Ptolemy collated and organised all the contemporary
thinking on astrology; he was not an innovator (Tester, 1987, p. 60).
Cornelius argues Ptolemy discarded the divinatory aspect of astrology to fit in with contemporary rational Stoic philosophy (Cornelius,
1994, p. 112).

Ptolemy's Tetrabiblos

Book One summarised the workings of the Sun and Moon and planets,
as well as some fixed stars. Stoics believed the same physical laws
applied throughout the universe, and that the planets affect all earthly
creatures in a predictable and orderly fashion. Herbs ruled by Venus,
for example, tend to heal the organs of generation which are themselves

ruled by Venus. Although Ptolemy does not mention herbs, he is very clear on the important relationship between astrology and medicine:

> concerning nativities and individual temperaments in general ...
> there are circumstances of no small importance and of no trifling
> character, which join to cause the special qualities of the native.
> (Robbins, 1940, p. 17, my translation.)

In Book Two he sets out his philosophical arguments for astrology "within the limits of natural reason" and how to interpret eclipses (Parker & Parker, 1983, p. 42). Ptolemy's Aristotelian-Stoic leanings are clearly shown: "It could very easily and very clearly be demonstrated ... power from the outer ether-like invisible nature is distributed over and penetrates all the wholly-changeable substances round the earth" (Tester, 1987, p. 64).

Book Three concerns horoscopy. Countering arguments that conception is really the beginning of life ($\alpha\rho\chi\eta$) and impossible to time for a horoscope, Ptolemy argued the moment of birth was the true beginning of life (*katarche*, $\kappa\alpha\tau\alpha\rho\chi\eta$), and that, according to Egyptian sources, the sign of the Moon at conception will be the ascendant at birth (Tester, 1987, p. 79).

Ptolemy wrote that: "The nature of the planet produces the forms and causes of the symptoms" (Robbins, 1940, p. 309). This is Ptolemy's "scientific" take on astrology and medicine. For example, Saturn is cooling and drying because it is the planet furthest away from the warmth of the Sun. For this reason, "Saturn makes men cold-bellied ... emaciated, weakly" (Tester, 1987, p. 63). Ptolemy believed the temperament of each man was determined by the state of the heaven at his birth (his horoscope). For example, the placement of Saturn in the ascendant of the birth-chart gave:

> swarthy complexioned, robust, black, curly hair, hirsute, moderate
> sized eyes, middle stature. Bodily temperament showing an excess
> of cold and moisture. (Robbins, 1940, p. 309.)

Ptolemy allowed that the environment, hereditary factors, and upbringing affected a person, but that the planetary effects were most powerful (the "machine of destiny" model, see p. 206). It was not a fatalistic doctrine, however, as man had the free will to predict what is foretold by the stars and adjust his conduct accordingly (Tester, 1987, p. 70).

Chapter 13 is concerned with "the quality of the soul" or how the planets affect the mind and how different planetary combinations may herald minor mental disorders, such as stupidity, extravagance, avarice, lewdness, etc. (Tester, 1987, p. 79). For example, mutable signs (Gemini, Virgo, Sagittarius, and Pisces) showed minds that were: "variable, versatile … volatile and unsteady, inclined to duplicity, amorous, wily, fond of music, careless, full of expedients and regretful" (Parker & Parker, 1983, p. 44). Fixed signs (Taurus, Leo Scorpio and Aquarius) were described as: "just, uncompromising, constant, firm of purpose, prudent, patient, industrious, strict, chaste, mindful of injuries, steady in pursuing its object, contentious, desirous of honour, seditious, avaricious and pertinacious" (Robbins, 1940, p. 355).

If Venus shows the soul, the native was "pleasant, good, cheerful, art-loving, decorous, compassionate and charming" (Robbins, 1940, p. 357), whereas Jupiter in poor condition (by sign and house) shows a soul with "wastefulness rather than magnanimity, superstition rather than respect for the gods, cowardice instead of modesty, conceit and not dignity, naivety and not kindness, the love of pleasure rather than the love of beauty" (Robbins, 1940, p. 347).

Chapter 14 of Book Three is concerned with serious mental disease, epilepsy, and insanity, which may be cured by diet and herbs if Jupiter is well-aspected or by prayer and sacrifices if Venus is shown (Tester, 1987, p. 79).

Book Four continues with the analysis of the horoscope, showing how wealth, rank, marriage, and profession are manifested. Mars, distant from Venus and Saturn, but near to Jupiter, will make people "pure and decorous in sexual intercourse, and incline them to natural usages only". Whereas if Mars were supported by Venus they "will become highly licentious and attempt to gratify their desires in every mode" (Parker & Parker, 1983, p. 45).

It is interesting that Galen and Ptolemy were colleagues and contemporaries. Their collected works were the standard texts on medicine and astrology until the Enlightenment in the seventeenth century. It may be argued, therefore, that the first century of our era marked the end of the ancient katarchic, magical worldview. As Galen recorded his medical theories, cementing his style of practice for the next 1,700 years, so did Ptolemy, with his calculation of the ephemerides, bring astrology down from the gods to the predictable and measurable and mundane.

Galen (129-c. 216 CE)

Galen was born in Pergamum (Bergama, western Turkey), a prosperous city in the Greek-speaking part of the Roman Empire. Pergamum was famous for its library (established in the third century BCE), which was one of the most important in the Western world after the Library of Alexandria. Plutarch wrote that it contained over 200,000 volumes. Galen studied medicine at the local temple sanctuary of Asclepius at Pergamum after his father dreamt the god said Galen should study the healing arts. Later, Galen studied in Alexandria, the greatest centre of learning at the time.

In 157 CE Galen became physician to the gladiators of Pergamum. He used diet, trauma medicine, and hygiene to heal their fractures and wounds. His skill in preventing sepsis and in wound-dressing meant he lost only two patients in four years; the previous holder of his office had lost sixteen (Nutton, 2013, p. 230).

Galen moved to Rome and became physician to the Emperor Commodus. During his lifetime, and for the next 1,200 years, Galen's methods and practice formed the basis of Western, Byzantine and Arabic medicine. Galen wrote over 500 treatises, approximately 10,000,000 words, of which 3,000,000 survive. His topics included anatomy, physiology, pathology, pharmacology, neurology, and philosophy. After the fall of the Roman Empire, his works written in Greek were preserved in the Byzantine Empire and, later, by Arab scholars in the Abbasid period (after 750 CE). Gradually, people in Europe lost the art of reading ancient Greek, so some of Galen's texts only exist in Arabic. After the fall of the Byzantine Empire (1453 CE) scholars came to Europe and brought his works with them.

Galen collected together all the current knowledge and practice of the medicine of his day, and added his own wide experience and learning. Nutton (2013, p. 219) claims Galen wrote extensive commentaries on the Hippocratic Corpus, dismissing those writings which did not support his (Galen's) theories of medicine and that furthermore Galen created, "an unerring Hippocrates in his own image" (Nutton, 2013, p. 219). Because he was so well-connected, as physician to the Emperor, Galen was able to establish himself as the medical expert of his time. Galen's works reflect his intelligent reasoning, detailed observation, and empirical testing of remedies and diseases (Nutton, 2013, p. 253).

Galen on anatomy

Human dissection was forbidden at that time, so Galen performed anatomical dissection on monkeys. Galen's anatomical findings and physiological theories held sway until Vesalius published his cadaver dissections in 1543. Vesalius' *De Humani Corporis Fabrica* was heavily influenced by Galen's work. Galen was the first to differentiate motor and sensory nerves and to discuss the concept of muscle tone. Galen also recognised the difference between arterial and venous blood; his theory on the circulation of the blood lasted until 1221 when Ibn al-Nafis wrote that blood circulated through the body with the heart acting like a pump. Galen's work with the gladiators of Pergamum gave him privileged access to anatomy through his study of their wounds, which he described as "windows into the body" (Nutton, 2013, p. 230).

Galen on medical practice

Nutton suggests part of Galen's undoubted success as a physician was his skills at prognosis, which he was keen to distinguish from prophecy and divination. He insisted each patient was to be treated as an individual: "one shoe does not fit all feet" (Nutton, 2013, p. 245). Galen used the Hippocratic system of dividing illness into stages and critical days (after Hippocrates' *Epidemics*).

Galen also promoted the four humours[1] and temperaments of the Hippocratic Corpus and the Hippocratic practice of bloodletting, which was unknown in Rome at that time. Galen related the properties of foods to the four humours, assigning them the qualities of heating and cooling, drying and moistening. Galen recommended a light diet and moderate exercise (Nutton, 2013, p. 246).

---

[1]Although it is unlikely Hippocrates subscribed to humoral theory, generally it is understood that his son-in-law Polybius was responsible for its inclusion in the Hippocratic corpus (Nutton, 2013, p. 246).

Galen on therapeutics

Although Galen wrote that Dioscorides' work was "the most perfect of treatises on materia medica" (Nutton, 2013, p. 244) Galen was more interested in developing his own theory of medicine. Galen analysed medicines from the perspective of their own qualities and the parts of the body affected by illness. For example, a phlegmagogue attracted phlegm and then expelled it from the body (Nutton, 2013, p. 249). Drug actions were classified as weak, obvious, strong, or massive. Galen further divided each category into small, moderate, and substantial in effect. Galen's pharmacopoeia contained 475 remedies, 161 of which he classified according to this system (Nutton, 2013, p. 251). Galen argued that each remedy was a mixture ($\kappa\rho\alpha\sigma\iota\varsigma$) and might be drying in the fourth degree and cold in the first. Dioscorides classified henbane as soporific in action, while Galen wrote it was cooling to the third degree and, furthermore, as the principal organ of coldness was the brain, henbane would cause dullness and confusion (Riddle, 1985, p. 171).

Galen, ever the pragmatist, believed that humble plants and herbs growing in the woods and fields beyond the city gates were more profitable to patients than exotic and complex mixtures sold by other doctors (Nutton, 2013, p. 245) as Culpeper was to write 1500 years later.

Galen on philosophy

Galen developed the Platonic theory that the soul was divided into three and he situated each part in an organ. The rational soul was found in the brain and was concerned with imagination, memory, recollection, knowledge, thought, consideration, voluntary motion, and sensation. The spiritual soul was found in the heart and was concerned with passions like anger, growing, and being alive. Galen believed that the passions were stronger than regular emotions and for that reason were more dangerous. The appetitive soul situated in the liver controlled the living forces in the body, especially the blood. It regulated the pleasures of the body and was moved by feelings of enjoyment. This was the more natural part of the soul and dealt with natural urges and survival instincts. Hence the soul contributed to the health of the body and strengthened the functional capacity of these three organs (Nutton, 2013, p. 239).

Galen adapted the theories of *pneuma*, which linked body and soul. Through the circulation of pneuma the soul interacted with the body and the organs interacted with one another. Galen located psychic pneuma in the brain and nervous system, and vital pneuma in the arterial system and heart. The liver, being the organ of digestion, broke down food and turned it into nutritious blood, which was transported in the veins to nourish the body. Venous blood mixed with pneuma in the heart to form vital spirit and circulated around the body. A small amount of this arterial blood went to the brain where it produced psychic pneuma, which circulated through the nervous system. Everything, plant, animal and man, had four natural faculties: attraction, assimilation, excretion, and growth. Thus, each part could attract, nourish, excrete, and grow and was in effect "a living universe" responding to changes and seeking what it needed to flourish; a vitalist approach (Nutton, 2013, p. 239).

Galen on psychology

Anger is an illness of the soul.

Ignorance an ugliness.

Illnesses of the body are generated by the corruption and disagreement of the things from which the body is constituted.

For health is the agreement and harmony of these things.

Ugliness is the opposite to fineness, and fineness in the body is due to the balance in its constitutional parts, ugliness is due to its unbalance.

The Soul's beauty comes from knowledge, its ugliness from ignorance. (Cited in Nutton, 2013, p. 161.)

John Gerard (c. 1545–1612)

Gerard was an English botanist and herbalist. He was the author of a large (1,484 pages) illustrated *Herball, or Generall Historie of Plantes*. First published in 1597, it was the most widely circulated botany book in English in the seventeenth century. Gerard's *Herbal* is largely based on Rembert Dodoens' *Cruydenboeck*, published in 1554, itself also highly popular (in Dutch, Latin, French, and other English translations).

Gerard was a high-ranking member of the barber surgeons company. He developed his garden in Holborn, which he often mentions in the *Herball*, and later published a catalogue of the plants he grew there. Gerard had a wide and influential network and people brought him seeds from the colonies of the New World. Gerard was the first to describe the potato in England, although he mistakenly gave its origin as Virginia and not South America. In 1586, the College of Physicians appointed Gerard curator of their physic garden, a position he held till 1604. George Baker (a friend and colleague) describes as follows this garden in his preface to the *Herball*: "all manner of strange trees, herbes, rootes, plants, floures and other such rare things, that it would make a man wonder, how one of his degree, not having the purse of a number, could ever accomplish the same" (Woodward, 1971, p. xi).

John Gerard was among a group of Renaissance natural historians, who sought to systematise natural history, re-working the writings of the ancients (Ogilvie, 2006, p. 6). The basis for Gerard's *Herball*, like those of Dodoens and other herbalists, was the *De Materia Medica* of Dioscorides. The botanical genus *Gerardia* was named after Gerard.

Gerard on Violet

The flowers and leaves of Violets are cold and moist.

The flowers are good for all inflammations, especially of the sides and lungs they take away the hoarseness of the chest ruggedness of the wind-pipe and jaws, allay the extreme heat of the kidneys and bladder, mitigate the fiery heat of burning agues, temper the sharpness of choler, and take away thirst.

There is an oile made of Violets which is likewise cold and moist. The same being anointed upon the testicles doth gently provoke sleep which is hindered by a hot and dry distemper; [the herb] mixed or laboured together in a wooden dish with the yolk of an egg, it is likewise good to be put into cooling clysters, and into poultices that cool and ease pain. The later physicians think it good to mix dry Violets with medicines that are to comfort and strengthen the heart.

The leaves of Violets inwardly taken do cool, moisten, and make the belly soluble. Being outwardly applied they mitigate all kind of hot inflammations. Dioscorides writes, that they be also applied to the fundament that is fallen out. Pliny says that Violets are as well used in garlands, as for smell, and are good against surfeting, heaviness of the head.

There is a syrup made of Violets and sugar, whereof three or four ounces taken at one time, soften the belly and purge choler.

The decoction of Violets is good again for hot fevers and the inflammation of the liver, and all other inward parts. Syrup of Violets is good against the inflammation of the lungs and breast, against the pleurisy and cough, against fevers and agues in young children,

The leaves of Violets are used in cooling plasters, oils, and comfortable cataplasms or poultices and are of greater efficacy among other herbs, as Mallows, and such like, clysters for the purposes aforesaid. (Gerard, 1636, p. 852.)

William Lilly (1602–1681)

Discretion, together with art. (Lilly, 1647, p. 397.)

It could be said that Lilly was the last famous and influential astrologer in England. Like Culpeper, he was a parliamentarian, although he had sympathy for the King Charles I. He wrote almanacs under the name *Merlinus Anglicus Junior*, making predictions of astrological phenomena as they affected politics. He was tremendously successful. In 1649 he sold nearly 30,000 copies of his almanac. Lilly correctly predicted Parliament's victory at the battle of Naseby in 1645 and the violent death of the King.

Lilly published *Christian Astrology* in 1647, the first astrology textbook in English. Lilly wrote his book in the spirit of Culpeper, making astrological and medical learning available to the ordinary people. Like Culpeper, Lilly saw medicine and astrology as one science. And like Ptolemy, Lilly collected together to extant knowledge of his day. There are 228 astrological works citied in his book, to which he added his own judgements. Lilly covers natal and horary astrology in the book, including decumbiture.

> I have with all uprightness and sincerity of heart, plainly and honestly delivered the Art, and have omitted nothing willingly ... verily the Method is my owne, it's no translation; yet I have conferred my own notes with Dariot, Bonatus, Ptolemy, Haly, Etzler, Dietericus, Naibod ... Agripa ... Argol. (Lilly, 1647, n.p.)

Lilly had a busy practice, his casebooks for 1644–66 show he saw around two thousand people a year. His clients were a mixture of servant girls and the great and the good. For the wealthy he charged £40 for a consultation. He also taught astrology. By 1662, his income was £500 per annum, a considerable sum (Parker & Parker, 1983, p. 155).

Later, Lilly moved into the country. Every Sunday he rode to Kingston for the day, as Ashmole recalls, "where the poorer sort flockt to him from several Parts" (Lilly, 1715, p. 102).

Lilly on divination

> [B]e humane, courteous, familiar to all, easie of access, afflict not the miserable with the terror of harsh judgement; in such cases let them know their hard fate by degrees … be modest, conversant with the learned, civil, sober man, covet not an estate; give freely to the poor, both money and judgement. (Lilly, 1647, Preface).

Nicholas Culpeper (1616–1654)

Culpeper was an English herbalist and astrologer, trained as an apothecary, who set up a pharmacy at Spitalfields, a location deliberately chosen to be outside the control of the City of London. After making a good marriage Culpeper was able to treat his patients for free. Like Dioscorides, Culpeper was a hands-on physician. He worked in the field, cataloguing medicinal herbs. Culpeper also examined patients rather than relying on urine diagnosis ("piss prophets"). His clinic was very busy. The College of Apothecaries tried to stop him practising, accusing him of witchcraft.

Culpeper fought on the parliamentary side at the battle of Newbury and carried out battlefield surgery. He was wounded and never fully recovered. Culpeper's radical politics encouraged him to break the monopoly of the College of Physicians. In 1649 he published and translated the *Pharmacopoeia Londinesis* from Latin to English to make it available to the ordinary reader. During the Civil War, the authority of the King and the Star Chamber was suspended, which meant a bonanza for publishing radical books that attacked the corrupt oligarchies. The following year he published *A Directory for Midwives*, a self-help guide of gynaecology and obstetrics. In 1652 he published *The English Physician* at a deliberately low price so everyone could afford it. *The English Physician* has never been out of print. His works include: *Pharmacopoeia Londinensis* (1649) a translation of the London Directory, reprinted in 1651 with a *Key to Galen and Hippocrates*. Later editions included

An Astrologo-Physical Discourse [Semeiotica Uranica] (1655). Other works: *Directory for Midwives* (1651); *The English Physician* (1652), later renamed *The Complete Herbal* (1653); *Galen's Art of Physic* (1652).

The English Physician

> I consulted with my two brothers, DR. REASON and DR. EXPERIENCE, and took a voyage to visit my mother NATURE, by whose advice, together with the help of DR. DILIGENCE, I at last obtained my desire; and, being warned by MR. HONESTY, a stranger in our daies, to publish it to the world, I have done it. (Culpeper, 1798, unnumbered page.)

Culpeper claimed this work surpassed the popular herbals of Gerard and Parkinson.

> Three hundred and sixty-nine medicines made of English Herbs ... Being an Astrologo-Physical Discourse of the vulgar Herbs of this Nation, containing a compleat method of Physic whereby a man may preserve his body in health or cure himself being sick with such things that grow in England, they being most fit for English bodies.
> Herein is also showed these seven things:
>
> 1. The way of making plaisters, oyntments, oil, pultisses, syrups, decoctions, julepes or waters, of all sorts of physical herbs.
> 2. What planet governeth every herb and tree that growth.
> 3. The time of gathering all herbs, both vulgarly and astrologically.
> 4. The way of drying and keeping the herbs all the year.
> 5. The way of keeping their juyces ready for use at all times.
> 6. The way of making and keeping all kinds of useful compounds made of herbs.
> 7. The way of mixing medicines according to the cause and mixture of the disese and part of the body afflicted.
> (Culpeper, 1798, p. 239)

Culpeper on Wormwood

> Wormwood is a herb of Mars. It is hot and dry in the first degree, viz. just as hot as your blood and no hotter. It remedies the evils

choler can inflict on the body of man by sympathy, it helps evils
Venus can inflict by antipathy; and it cleanseth the blood of choler.
It provokes urine, helps surfeits, swellings in the belly; it causeth an
appetite to meat, because Mars rules the attractive faculty in man;
the Sun never shone on a better herb for jaundice than this. Wormwood being a herb of Mars, is the perfect remedy for the bitings of
mice and rats. Mushrooms are under the dominium of Saturn, if
anyone has poisoned himself by eating them, Wormwood a herb
of Mars cures him, because Mars is exalted in Capricorn the house
of Saturn, and this it doth by sympathy. Wheals, pushes, black and
blue spots, coming either by bruises or beatings, Wormwood, the
herb of Mars helps. Mars eradicates all diseases in the throat by his
herbs (of which Wormwood is one) and this by antipathy. The eyes
are under the luminaries: the right eye of a man, the left eye of a
woman, the Sun claims dominion over, the left eye of man and the
right of woman, are the privilege of the Moon: wormwood, a herb
of Mars cures both. (Culpeper, 1798, p. 239)

Culpeper as a radical

I am confident that there be those in this Nation who have wit
enough to know that the *Papists* and *College of Physitians* will not
suffer *Divinity* and *Physick* to be printed in our mother tongue, both
upon one and the same grounds, and both colour it over with the
same excuses. (Culpeper, 1649, p. 4.)

As a Parliamentarian, Culpeper was against the monopoly of the ruling
classes, including the College of Physicians, who were monarchists
supporting the doomed King Charles I. His intention in translating the
medical works into English was to make available medical knowledge,
particularly of common herbs and roots to the unlicensed practitioners
and lay people who could not afford the price of a registered physician.
Furthermore, Culpeper believed these same physicians, hiding behind
their social standing and knowledge of Latin, were dangerous as well
as costly.

The ordinary people had no other remedies than the herbs that grew
in the byways of rural England. Culpeper's work encouraged the lay
person to reject the occasionally noxious mixtures of the apothecaries
and instead use fresh herbs, dietary medicine, and star lore to heal
themselves.

I think Culpeper would be unsurprised to see medicine in the twenty-first century beholden to big pharma, just as in the seventeenth century it was to the College of Physicians.[2]

Maud Grieve (1858–1941)

Maud Grieve was a herbalist, plants-woman, and writer. In October 1914 the Board of Agriculture published Bulletin No. 288, *The Cultivation & Collection of Medicinal plants in England,* to deal with the inadequate supplies of medicinal herbs that had previously been imported. Among those required were the narcotics: Henbane, Foxgloves, Deadly Nightshade and Monkshood. Mrs Grieve converted her nursery to the cultivation of medicinal herbs and began her life's work: the writing of herbal monographs. She founded the National Herb Growing Association (1914–17) and became president of the British Guild of Herb Growers (est. 1918). She opened The Whins Medicinal and Commercial Herb School during the 1914–1918 war. Mrs Grieve's monographs on individual herbs were collected and edited by Hilda Leyel, a herbalist. They became *A Modern Herbal,* published in 1931. Her book contains instructions for the growing, preparation, and dosages of over 300 herbs, together with references and recipes from Dioscorides, Gerard, and Culpeper, amongst others.

Alan Leo (1860–1917)

Alan Leo, known as "the father of modern astrology" is credited with almost singlehandedly saving and reinventing astrology for the modern age in Europe and America, following its decline at the end of the seventeenth century. A committed theosophist, Leo introduced spiritual ideas such as reincarnation and karma into his work. Using the Theosophical Society's large international network, Leo was able to spread his new vision of modern astrology worldwide.

Leo was taught astrology by an astrological herbalist in Nottingham at the age of eighteen. At twenty-two he discovered the idea of

---

[2]Culpeper was especially against the importation and use of costly, exotic remedies from the new colonies, which he saw as a ruse to extract even larger fees from long-suffering patients. A parallel can be drawn with the use of sophisticated, exorbitant pharmaceuticals where simpler remedies would work just as well (Culpeper, 1649, p. 3).

reincarnation and karma, and by twenty-eight he was deep into the study of natal astrology. In 1889 he became a theosophist and started the *Astrologer's Magazine* with F.W. Lacey. In 1895 he started a new magazine, *Modern Astrology*, writing that: "The time has come to modernize the ancient system of Astrology" (Curry, 1992, p. 134). Leo then founded an astrological society in 1896, the first of several.

In 1914 Leo was charged under the Vagrancy Act for "professing to tell fortunes". He was found not guilty, but this threat of prosecution made him determined to replace the planetary "influences" of what he regarded as "the fatalistic school of materialistic Astrology" (Leo, 1911, p. 25) with psychological "tendencies", in keeping with his slogan, "Character is Destiny" (Curry, 1992, p. 150). In 1914 he founded the Astrological Lodge of the Theosophical Society, which still exists, teaching astrology. All contemporary astrology organisations are derived from the Astrological Lodge, including the Company of Astrologers.

The Company of Astrologers was founded by Maggie Hyde, Geoffrey Cornelius, and Gordon Watson in 1983.[3] It is the home of astrology as divination and seeks to establish a modern, craft-based discipline of traditional astrology that acknowledges insights from philosophy and psychotherapy, as well as revisioning horoscopy in the light of divination (*katarche*, see p. 206).

Hilda Leyel (1880–1957)

Mrs Leyel studied the work of the herbalist Nicholas Culpeper and his predecessors. In 1926 she wrote *The Magic of Herbs* and in 1927 she opened Culpeper House in Baker Street, selling herbal medicines, foods, and cosmetics. Mrs Leyel founded the Society of Herbalists (later, the Herb Society, which continues to this day) a non-profit-making organization for the study and practice of herbal medicine. In 1941 the Pharmacy and Medicines Bill threatened to outlaw the practice of herbalism in England. Mrs Leyel was well-connected, and with the support of powerful friends managed to have the bill amended to enable patients to obtain treatment on joining the Society of Herbalists.

---

[3]Graeme Tobyn, Joanna Watters, and I studied and lectured at the Company of Astrologers.

PART TWO

THE PRACTICE

"Medicine rests upon four pillars—philosophy, astronomy, alchemy, and ethics. The first pillar is the philosophical knowledge of earth and water; the second, astronomy, supplies its full understanding of that which is of fiery and airy nature; the third is an adequate explanation of the properties of all the four elements—that is to say, of the whole cosmos—and an introduction into the art of their transformations; and finally, the fourth shows the physician those virtues which must stay with him up until his death, and it should support and complete the three other pillars."

Paracelsus

This section has two parts; the first is the diagnosis and treatment of sickness through astrology, called Decumbiture, the second is the maintenance of health through discovering the Temperament of the body and working with its strengths and minimizing its weaknesses.

The decumbiture method

A physician without astrology is like a pudding without fat.
(Culpeper, 1651a, p. 75.)

Decumbiture is Latin for "concerning the time of lying down". A decumbiture chart was made for the time a person felt so sick they took to their bed. However, it was and can be used for the time a person contacts the practitioner (in Lilly's day, when they brought the urine to be examined), or I use it for when the client first comes to see me, their first appointment.[1]

Decumbiture is a particular form of astrology, horary astrology, the astrology of asking questions. The rules are different from those of natal horoscopy, and the instructions on how to proceed are clear and precise.

A decumbiture is a representation or symbol of the illness, the patient, the practitioner, the medicine or treatment indicated, and the outcome. It provides the practitioner with timing measures for when best to perform a treatment, and when to expect healing crises and resolution of the issue. It also, most importantly, shows the best way the practitioner can help the patient, or, to use Cornelius' language, how to invoke the

---

[1]Lilly discusses the options a practitioner has when choosing the best time to use to erect a decumbiture chart in *Christian Astrology* (1647, p. 270).

197

patient's daemon for healing to occur (Cornelius, 1994, p. 193). As such, the decumbiture is not a fated map of destiny along Ptolemaic lines (the machine of destiny), but an active divination which shows through symbols how best the situation might be addressed.

Decumbiture works from a physical level; it will show the herbs and diet needed to improve conditions, but it will also show emotional and mental factors, which might have contributed to the condition, and I believe it shows spiritual energies at work that are affecting the case.

In this sense, a decumbiture can be said to represent a wholistic picture of the patient as they present to the practitioner, and the practitioner as they prepare to work with the patient. It is, in effect, a hermeneutic approach which "is not anti-science, but which counters 'scientism' that is, the inappropriate extension of scientific method to phenomena and domains of experience which cannot be reduced to objective and positive assertions of a literal nature" (Cornelius, 1994, p. xxi).

Horary astrology talks about "the radicality of the chart"; by this it means, do the symbols reveal an important truth about the matter? And are the symbols appropriate and readable within the limits of the horary approach? (Cornelius, 1994, p. 29.) Signs and causes are often confused as one and the same, but the planets do not *cause* a disease, they offer a symbolic representation to the astrologer from which she or he can move and act to improve the health of the patient, with the patient's co-operation and input. The astrologer cannot be separated from their clients, nor can the herbalist from their patient.[2]

Gordon Watson wrote on process in horary, which I believe can be applied to the decumbiture chart. He saw four categories of "takes" or observations from a chart. First, the astrological symbols had to fit the subject, a hot illness needs to be shown by hot planets and signs, for example. Second, the subject matter must limit the astrologer's remit; if it is a question about health, then other subjects are peripheral to the question.[3] Third, the chart has a meaningful context; the herbalist or

[2]An interesting example in Chinese medicine was expounded by Giovanni Maciocia in a YouTube discussion of *gui*. He declared that acupuncture was very individual, and the treatment depended on how the practitioner was at the moment of treatment, that is, how his *shen* was at that time would influence the success or otherwise of the treatment (Maciocia, 2015, 32'22").

[3]Health, as a complex, multi-layered question, can have its roots in other subject areas: relationships, money, housing, etc. However, the primary focus should be on the subject-matter—the health of the enquirer.

astrologer is a significant element of the context in which the chart is interpreted, for there is no objectivity or neutrality in the interpretation.[4] Finally, there is the herbalist's creative imagination, which encompasses the first three points and adds an extra dimension: a mixture of intuitive knowing, past experience and present-moment perceptions, which all contribute towards making the judgement (Watson, in Cornelius, 1994, p. 220).

By understanding both the astrological symbols (planets, signs, and houses), which illustrate and elucidate their story, the questioner (querent) is moved to act and transform both their behaviour and their understanding of their situation. This insight marks the beginning of their healing journey. The level at which the symbols are interpreted depends on the emotional and spiritual development of both the herbalist and the patient. For example, choler may be seen simply as heat, or may represent a spiritual longing for action and transformation which is unrecognised or unfulfilled.

Within the decumbiture there lies the possibility for negative interpretations, highlighting the importance of the strictures (rules preventing the reading of a chart), which prevent misfortune (or a bad diagnosis). It is not always appropriate to use astrology if a stricture arises in the decumbiture; the herbalist or astrologer is bound to respect this and withdraw. This does not mean the patient cannot be treated, but it does mean that astrology is of limited use in this instance. Strictures represent a red flag moment for medical astrology.

It follows then, that *katarche* in the form of the decumbiture empowers the patient, who asks the question of the herbalist with great sincerity and after much soul-searching, and orientates the herbalist to the proper conduct with regard to the herbalist themselves, as a practitioner, and towards the client and the symbolism the chart offers them. By means of rules (strictures) bad or poor divination is prevented (for example, when a chart shows a retrograde Mercury, insisting that the chart is

---

[4] I remember seeing this when training as a herbalist: people attracted certain types of patients. Although patients were assigned on a random basis, nevertheless it appeared a greater logic was operating and we would receive patients who could teach us about ourselves as well as about herbal medicine. Practitioners will also recognise the phenomenon of how, when personally dealing with an issue, clients will come with the same issue. This happens on such a regular basis as to be a truism. It underlines the fact that the practitioner is not an objective bystander, but a subjective participant in the healing relationship, and their knowledge, interpretations, and experience colour the diagnosis and treatment.

unsafe to judge, or that not everything has been revealed which is germane to the question). The decumbiture offers further gifts as it then shows the nature of healing (herbs or other modalities) and gives timing measures, which show the best time to treat the patient, and how the patient can facilitate their own healing process, because the truth is that healing doesn't happen "out there", but within a relationship of transformation between practitioner and client, in which both are changed.

Glossary of astrological terms

Almuten

A planet which, because of the house it is in, its dignities, fortitudes, and aspects (see Ptolemy's Table of Planetary Dignities in Appendix 2), is the most important planet in either the whole chart or in a house. For the purposes of calculating the temperament, it is the almuten of the whole chart that is added in the table. Most astrological software will calculate the almuten.

Angles

The angles in both a horary and a natal chart refer to the ascendant and descendant, and the IC (*imum coeli*, "bottom of the sky") and MC (*medium coeli*, "middle of the sky"). The ascendant is the first house, the descendant exactly opposite, the seventh house, the MC the tenth house and the IC exactly opposite is the fourth house.

Ascendant

Also called the *rising sign*. This is the sign which was rising in the heavens at the time the chart was cast. The *degree rising* is the degree of the sign which marks the ascendant. In horary astrology, if the degree rising is less than 3° it is said it is too early to make a judgement, while if the degree rising is more than 27° it is said it is too late to make a judgement. In natal astrology, the ascendant is the face people see, not necessarily who a person is on the inside, but the persona or public face. In horary astrology, the ascendant or rising sign shows the person asking the question, the *querent* (see p. 208 for a more detailed discussion). In both horary and aatal astrology, the ascendant or rising sign (and any planets on the ascendant or in the first house) should show the physical appearance of the person. The correlation between the rising sign and appearance is the first test of *radicality* (see below, p. 209).

Aspects

Because the horoscope is a circle, there is a geometrical relationship between the planets in a chart. Aspects are positive or negative. If two planets are moving towards an aspect they are said to be *applying*. When the planets are moving away from an aspect they are said to be *separating* (see below, p. 210). Applying aspects are stronger (the thing has yet to happen) than separating aspects (the thing has happened, and its effects are moving away).

Conjunction

A planet is situated next to another (see *orb* for how close). This may be positive or negative.

Cazimi

If a planet is within 17 minutes (not degrees) of a conjunction of the Sun, traditionally it is said to be very strong. I have not found much evidence for this.

Combustion

When a planet is within 8.5° of a conjunction of the Sun, it is said to be combust, that is, its energy is burned up by the rays of the Sun and it has little power. If the ruler of the ascendant is combust, then the question may not be answered or the querent will take no notice of the judgement. In either case it is unwise to proceed.

Sun, Moon conjunction (New Moon)

This is seen as a malefic sign, especially if the Moon is applying to the Sun. But judgement can be made.

Sunbeams

When a planet is within 17° of the sun it is under sunbeams. This weakens the planet but less so than *combustion* (see above). For example, if the querent is shown by a combust planet (within 8.5° of the Sun) and the planet is applying to the Sun, the disease is serious. If the planet is combust but separating, that is, moving away, then the person was seriously ill but will now recover. If the planet is under sunbeams, they are ill, but not seriously, and even less so if the planet is separating from the Sun.

Opposition

When a planet is 180° apart from another planet, in the sign diametrically opposite. For example, one planet in Aries, the other in Libra. Oppositions show stress and difficulty, opposition in fact. This is a bad aspect.

Quincunx

Where planets are 150° apart, for example: a planet in Aries will be quincunx one in Virgo. This is an aspect of difficulty and is mostly used in decumbiture to give more information about the sickness.

Square

A planet is 45° from another planet. For example, one planet in Aries and another in either Cancer or Capricorn. Again, this is an aspect of stress, but less stressful than an opposition, and shows that things may work out, but with difficulty. This is a bad aspect.

Sextile

This is when a planet is 60° from another, a harmonious aspect. An Aries planet will be sextile to a Gemini planet and an Aquarian planet. The sextile is less beneficial than a trine, but shows a good outcome, nevertheless.

Semi-sextile

This is a minor aspect of 30°. I rarely use these aspects except when it is the final aspect the Moon makes before leaving a sign (see *void of course Moon*).

Trine

This is when a planet is 90° from another. They will be in the same element and so harmoniously combined. An Aries planet will be trine another in Leo and Sagittarius (both Fire signs). This is a good aspect of harmony and bodes well for the question or questioner.

Benefic and malevolent planets

Benefic (helpful and positive) planets are Jupiter and Venus and the Sun. Malefic (unhelpful and harmful) planets are Mars and Saturn in traditional astrology, but I would also include the three trans-Saturnian planets (Uranus, Neptune and Pluto) as generally malefic, particularly in the short-term. From a long-term perspective, the trans-Saturnian planets often bring positive changes, but they show stress and difficulty.

Condition of a planet

Planets can be strong or weak (their *condition*) depending upon which sign and house they are in. The table of essential dignities in Appendix 2 shows in which signs the planets are in dignity, exaltation, which signs they rule, and where they are in detriment and fall.

Co-ruler

The trans-Saturnian planets have been assigned signs and are known as their co-rulers. Pluto is the co-ruler of Scorpio, Neptune of Pisces, and Uranus of Aquarius. When looking at a chart take whichever of the co-rulers to signify the querent or quesited that best describes the situation or person.

Co-significator

The Moon is always co-significator in a horary. If the ruler of the ascendant and the ruler of the sixth are the same planet, for example, the ascendant is Taurus and the sixth house is Libra, then the significator of both houses would be Venus. In such a case use the Moon as significator of the querent. I always look at the Moon as co-significator of the querent; it provides more detail, or another angle, in understanding what is happening in a chart.

Crisis days

In a decumbiture to plot the acute crisis days, take the sign and degree of the Moon and plot forwards until the Moon is square the decumbiture Moon. For example, in a decumbiture if the Moon is at 10° Taurus the first crisis day will be when the Moon is at 10° Leo (square aspect); the second crisis at 10° Scorpio (opposition aspect); and the third and final at 10° Aquarius (square aspect). These crisis days are generally around seven days apart. In a chronic crisis chart, use the sign and degree of the Sun from the decumbiture and again, plot the Sun square, opposite, and square again the decumbiture Sun.

Cusp

This is the line which separates one house from another. Planets are seen to be on the cusp when they are near to this dividing line. Planets on the cusp draw attention to the next house. Some astrologers put these planets into the next house. But, as a wise Taurean once said, they are where they are, and so I read them as being in the house which they are in. When looking for the planetary ruler of a house, the sign which is on the cusp of that house and the planet which rules that sign is said to be the ruler of the house. For example, if the cusp of the sixth house is Aries, Aries is ruled by Mars, so Mars is said to be the ruler of the sixth house. Even though Mars may be in any house of the horoscope, it has dominion over the sixth house in this case. And as we will discover in the decumbiture method, the planet ruling the sixth will show the nature of the sickness.

Descendant

See *angles*, above.

Detriment

The sign in which a planet is weak, for example Venus is in detriment in Aries, and Mars in Taurus. (See the Table of Dignities in Appendix 2 for the full list.)

THE DECUMBITURE METHOD   205

Disposes/dispositor

This is where one planet has influence over the sign another planet is in. For example, if the Moon is in Gemini, Mercury, ruler of Gemini, is said to dispose the Moon. The astrologer then looks to the condition of Mercury in the chart which will influence the expression of the Moon in Gemini.

Decumbiture

A chart drawn up for either the time of falling sick, the first contact of the patient, or the time of the first appointment.

Ephemeris

From the Greek (ημερα, *hemera*) meaning "day". It is a book which lists where all the planets are at a given time. You can get a fifty-year ephemeris, a hundred-year ephemeris, or a yearly one, which is particularly useful as it gives the exact times when planets are in aspect, which is useful for calculating crisis days.[5]

Fall

The sign in which a planet is weakest. For example, Mars in Cancer and Venus in Virgo. (See the Table of Dignities in Appendix 2 for the full list.)

Horary astrology

The astrology of questions.

Houses

The chart is divided into twelve houses counting from the eastern horizon or ascendant (nine o'clock position on a clock face). There are various systems for calculating the houses (although the ascendant

---

[5]For example: *Raphael's Astronomical Ephemeris of the Planet's Places*. Published each year by Foulsham in Marlow, Buckinghamshire.

remains constant in all of them). The majority of astrologers use the Placidus house system, and Regiomontanus (used by Lilly) is also popular; it is a question of the preference of the astrologer. Equal house is not recommended for horary but can be used in natal astrology. Free online calculations will generally be in Placidus. If you buy a program such as *Solar Fire* or use Zetsev.com (which is free) you can choose which house system you want the chart to be calculated in.

IC

See *angles*, above.

Judicial and intercidental days

In the decumbiture method, timing measures, the judicial day is when the Moon (or Sun in a chronic chart) has moved one complete sign from where it was in the decumbiture chart, for example from 15° Aries to 15° Taurus. The date and time that the Moon reaches 15° Taurus in our example is the first judicial day. When the Moon reaches 15° Gemini that is the first intercidental day. There are four judicial and four inter-cidental days in a lunar month. The same applies to solar charts for chronic conditions.

Katarche

From the Greek (*κατα αρχη*), "from the beginning". It describes a type of astrology concerned with beginnings; horary astrology and its sub-section, decumbiture. *Katarche* describes the relationship between the person asking the question, the subject matter of the question, and the person who is answering the question in terms of a divinatory process. Horary does not really ask what will happen, but more how should I proceed from here? This contrasts with natal astrology, which depicts the planets at the time of birth as a symbolic representation of an indi-vidual's character, life path, and (possibly) destiny. Natal astrology can suffer the Ptolemaic affliction of the "machine of destiny" model, which suggests it is all written and predestined. Horary and decumbi-ture, by contrast, allow for interpretation of the next step needed to complete or achieve a desired outcome (or the barriers and obstacles to achieving it).

Lord of the hour and day

As discussed above, each day of the week is assigned its own planet: Moon, Monday; Mars, Tuesday, etc. Similarly, each hour is assigned its own planet; the first hour after sunrise is ruled by the same planet as rules the day; Moon for Monday, Mars for Tuesday, etc., and the eighth hour is also ruled by the planet of the day (as all seven traditional planets have had one hour each). It is useful to note the *planetary day and hour* to see the influences at work in the decumbiture.

Lunar cycle

This is the length of time it takes the moon to travel around the whole zodiac. It is usually around 28.3 days long.

Midheaven

See *angles*, above.

Moon

See p. 221 for importance of, and timing measures.

Mute signs

These are Cancer, Scorpio, and Pisces. If either the ascendant, Moon, or rulers of the querent or quesited are in mute signs, this can show secrecy or something which is not being revealed. It is similar to Mercury retrograde (see *retrograde*).

Mutual reception

See also *disposition*. This is where the planets ruling each other's sign change places (but keep their degrees). For example, Moon in Capricorn and Saturn in Cancer. The planets can exchange places, which may make some action by the *querent* possible. Appleby writes that mutual reception "promises the assistance of some third party, or gives an escape route from a difficult situation" (Appleby, 1985, p. 35).

Orb, or orbs of aspect

As said above, *applying aspects* are strongest and show what is going to happen, especially with the Moon. I use small orbs of 3° applying to an aspect. For example, Mercury in Taurus applying to a square (90°) of Jupiter in Leo. If Mercury is at 20° Taurus and Jupiter is between 17–20° Leo, I will say they are in square. The Moon, as discussed above, is allowed all aspects until she changes sign, but the closer the aspect (the smaller the orb) the quicker and stronger the effect.

Part of fortune and other Arabic parts

Sometimes also called *lots*. The part of fortune shows help in any situation or a more positive outcome than the planets might suggest, should the Moon or any other significators aspect it. The part of fortune is calculated by adding the degree of the ascendant to the Moon and subtracting the Sun. It is written in the chart as an X in a circle. Start counting at 0° Aries. So, if the ascendant is 10° Taurus that is (30+10) plus the Moon at say, 15° Gemini (30+30+15) less the Sun at 8° Cancer (30+30+30+8). 40+65–98=7 so the part of fortune (or *fortuna*) is 7° Aries. There are many Arabic parts. The part of sickness = ascendant + Mars – Saturn, written as an *S* in a circle. Part of death, ascendant + eighth cusp – Moon, written as a *D* in a circle. There are also parts of marriage, inheritance, accidents, and many more. (See Zoller, 1989.)

Peregrine

When a planet has no strength or dignity of any kind (see Appendix 2 for tables of dignity). A planet is peregrine when it is unable to influence events and is powerless.

Primary significator

These are the querent and the quesited. (See also *secondary significator* and *co-significator*.)

Querent

The person asking the question, which is shown by the ascendant in a decumbiture and the ruler of the ascendant becomes the significator (symbol) of the querent.

Quesited

The question asked. In the case of sickness this will be the ruler of the sixth house of sickness.

Radicality

This refers to the judgement of the horary astrologer as to whether the chart describes the situation and the chart has passed the necessary tests to be safe to judge. Tests of radicality include:

1. Is the rising sign less than 3° or more than 27° (see *ascendant*).
2. Is the Moon void of course; that is, will the Moon make any more aspects before it changes sign. A judgement of sorts can be made with a void of course moon (VC for short) because it signifies that nothing will come of the matter. So, if the question is, "will I get this job, or do I have a serious illness?" the answer, "nothing will come of the matter" gives a no. Conversely, if the question is, "am I pregnant?" the same answer, "nothing will come of the matter" applies; in this case, no you are not pregnant.
3. Via combusta: this is between 15° Libra and 15° Scorpio. If the ascendant or Moon is between these degrees, the chart is not safe to judge, except if they fall on the fixed star Spica, which is benefic. Personally, I tend to disregard this, but nevertheless proceed with caution.
4. Saturn: if found conjunct the ascendant or in the first house it is said to damage the question, while a retrograde Saturn is said to destroy the question. Derek Appleby observed that "the matter rarely ends well … and some misfortune intervenes to render the original questions irrelevant" (Appleby, 1985, p. 15). If Saturn is found in the seventh house of the astrologer, it can show it is not safe to make a judgement. For the purposes of medical astrology, I would then put down the chart and prescribe and treat without using astrology.

Retrograde

This refers to the apparent (but not real) phenomenon of a planet moving backwards in the heavens. It is shown on a horoscope by a *Px* sign. All planets except the Sun and Moon turn retrograde. Mercury retrogrades around three times a year, Venus and Mars maybe twice a year, for about three weeks. The slower moving planets, Jupiter to

Pluto, may be retrograde for many months at a time. When a planet is retrograde this signifies its energies are less accessible or that, especially in the case of Mercury, information is hidden or lost and there may be confusion about what is happening. Traditional horary astrology judges that when one of the significators in a chart is retrograde, the chart is not safe to judge. However, I have not found this to be so, rather, it shows there is more information to be revealed and that any judgement should be tentative or provisional. When the querent is shown by a retrograde planet, they may be concealing or unaware of vital information, unconscious forces may be at work, or, simply, that more will be revealed later on.

A retrograde planet in a natal chart often shows that the area of life symbolised by that planet, and its sign and house, are hard to access or confusing in some way, that there is difficulty in this area. It may be the energy is turned inwards, and, for example in the case of a retrograde natal Mercury, the inner life of the mind is richer than there are words to describe. Similarly, retrograde Mercury may show problems of expression (such as stuttering) or intellectual challenges.

Ruler

Also known as the *lord* or *ruling planet*. The ruler of a sign is the planet that has the strongest dignity in the sign. Mars rules Aries, Jupiter rules Sagittarius, Mercury rules Gemini. A planet found in the sign it rules is very strong (see Appendix 2 for the table of essential dignities).

Secondary significators

These will be any planets in the house of the quesited (in the case of health, the sixth house; for operations, any planets in the eighth; for hospitals, planets in the twelfth, etc.) See also *primary significator* and *co-significator*.

Separating and applying aspects

When one planet is moving towards another it is said to be applying (or in an applying aspect). When one planet is moving away from another planet, it is said to be separating. Aspects which are applying are more powerful than those which are separating, because the former is building-up to make contact, while the latter has made contact and is moving away. The Moon has special significance in separating and applying aspects. It is the fastest moving planet in the horoscope. Separating aspects of the Moon show what has recently happened, applying aspects of the Moon show what is going to happen. If there are no applying aspects (see *void of course Moon*) then nothing is going to happen. In decumbiture, the Moon's last separating aspect usually shows how the illness came about, or at least those factors which contributed to its genesis. The Moon's next applying aspect shows what will happen next, for good or ill. (See *benefic and malefic planets*.)

Significator

The planet which rules the house of the quesited and the querent. (See *primary significator*, *secondary significator* and *co-significator*.)

Strictures

These are the rules that traditionally prevent the judgement of a horary or decumbiture chart, for example, an early or late degree rising, a void of course moon, etc. (See *radicality*, above.) It is the art of the astrologer to determine whether to adhere to the strictures if they occur (for example, a retrograde Mercury, which occurs three times a year for several weeks at a time, and would make practising medical astrology very difficult). To begin with, I suggest observing them and then with experience to decide whether they should be disregarded.

Sympathy and antipathy

Treating by sympathy is to treat a disease of Venus with Venus herbs. Treating by antipathy is to treat a disease of Venus with herbs of Saturn (as Saturn is antipathetical to Venus). Ideally, treat by sympathy (to strengthen nature). However, it may be necessary to add antipathetical herbs to stop a debilitating symptom, for example, using a herb of Saturn to stop haemorrhage, while treating the underlying cause sympathetically.

Timing measures

Using the Moon (acute) or the Sun (chronic) to chart the progress of an illness, predict *crisis days* and good days for treatments (*judicial and intercidental*).

Void of course

This is when the Moon or any other planet will not make any further aspects before it changes sign. Some astrologers include among aspects the Moon's nodes and the *part of fortune*. I generally only judge aspects to planets when determining if a planet is *void of course*.

The decumbiture method

Traditionally, as mentioned earlier, the practitioner took the time of taking to one's bed to set up the chart, or when a urine sample was brought to the practitioner. In my practice, I use the time the appointment is made, unless there was a medical crisis that can be timed accurately.

A chart or horoscope may look complicated, but it is just a diagram of the relative position of the signs and planets of the zodiac at a particular time using particular tables. It is not an exact replica of the solar system. It helps to see it as the face of a clock which is divided into twelve sections, each representing the signs of the zodiac from Aries to Pisces. One of these signs rises over the eastern horizon; this is called the ascendant or first house and is drawn at nine o'clock on the birth chart. Charts these days are usually calculated by computer (free chart casting is available on several sites online).[6] By putting in the co-ordinates of the place, and the time and day of the question, a chart will be calculated. The chart will be a circle divided into twelve sections of unequal size. Each of these divisions is a house and will have a degree and sign, for example 20° Aries. This will give you the house cusp, the planet ruling the house cusp (in our example Mars will rule the house cusp as it is the ruler of Aries), and the degree of the cusp, which is used in the ascendant only to check for radicality, see below.

---

[6]Free sites include: www.zaytsev.com (this calculates the almuten, which is needed for temperament calculation), and www.astro.com. The software program most often used is *Solar Fire*, available from www.londonastrology.com.

Cast the chart, then decide if the chart is radical and capable of judgement.

Deciding radicality

The degree rising, if it is less than 3°, it can be said it is too soon to make a judgement on the matter. If it is more than 27°, then the matter has progressed to a stage where it is too late to make a judgement. These strictures can sometimes be worked around if the rest of the chart is radical. Lilly says this stricture can be ignored if the querent is very young and his complexion and body shape agrees with the quality of the sign ascending. If the degree is late the chart can be judged, according to Lilly, if the patient has the same age as the degree ascending (Lilly, 1647, p. 122).

The position of the Moon. If the Moon is not going to make any aspects before it changes sign, it is said to be void of course and the judgement is "nothing will come of the matter". This a judgement of sorts, because if the question is, "do I have cancer?", then the answer will be "nothing will come of the matter", meaning no. Lilly argues that sometimes a void of course Moon chart can be judged, when the Moon is in Taurus, Cancer, Sagittarius, or Pisces (Lilly, 1647, p. 122). The Moon is pivotal in decumbiture, as she will show what has happened, through previous aspects she has made, and what will happen, through her next aspect, and all the aspects she makes before she changes signs.

If the moon is between 15° Libra and 15° Scorpio she is said to be in the *via combusta* and the chart is not safe to judge. Again, sometimes this stricture can be worked around, but it is a red flag to take great care.

If Saturn is in the first house it destroys the question; "the matter of the question seldom or never comes to good" (Lilly, 1647, p. 122). Likewise, if Saturn is in the seventh house, it shows the judgement of the astrologer is unsound and the practitioner will not help the questioner.

If the lord (ruler) of the ascendant is combust (conjunct the Sun) then the question and questioner will not heed the advice of the practitioner (Lilly, 1647, p. 123). If the lord of the seventh is unfortunate or in its fall, the judgement of the practitioner will be unsound.

If Mercury is retrograde then the chart is not safe to judge, as either the judgement of the practitioner is faulty or there is something which is hidden or not being said. Again, I have worked with charts with a retrograde Mercury, and I usually find that something is revealed later that throws more light on the issue. So, with a retrograde Mercury, use discretion.

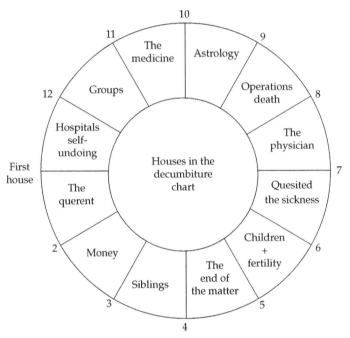

Figure 1. Houses in the decumbiture chart.

Working with a chart

The ascendant

The first test of radicality (does the chart speak of the case) is that the patient should physically resemble the ascendant. A small, petite patient is unlikely to be shown by planets and sign which tend to size: Jupiter, Pisces, Sagittarius, etc. A patient shown by Cancer rising will walk into the room hesitantly; one shown by Leo will be warm; by Libra, should talk a lot; Aries, a bit irritable, and so on. Obviously, people are not caricatures of the signs, but they should be recognisable. A very talkative patient shown by Scorpio is as unlikely as a quiet Gemini. If the ascendant seems not to make sense, look for planets in the first house. For example, Aries rising with Saturn in the first house will probably not come across as fiery, because Saturn (melancholic and a malefic) will crush the fire, but they may well be argumentative (Aries) and negative (Saturn) or passive-aggressive (Aries and Saturn).

If you see clients, it is a very fruitful exercise to go back and cast the decumbiture for those you know. Note the time of their first appointment and match their ascendant to what you remember of how they looked and behaved when you first met them. Think about how they dressed, did they arrive early or late, could they find your place? (Aquarians and Pisces are notorious for lateness, Librans for getting lost.) How did they come across, was their story rambling and hard to follow? (Water or sometimes Air.) Did you have to prise information out of them? (Scorpio, Neptune or Pluto on the ascendant.) Did they pay you effortlessly? (Leo.) Quibble about the bill? (Saturn or Capricorn or Earth.) Or forget their purse? (Gemini.) The way to work with this material is to collect as many examples as you can and then test the theories to see how they work out in practice.

The sickness

This is shown by the sixth house and the planet which rules the sign on the cusp of the sixth house. For example, if the sixth house is ruled by Gemini, the ruling planet will be Mercury, which rules Gemini. Look for where Mercury is placed in the chart and this may give clues as to reasons for being sick. For example, if the ruler of the sixth is in the tenth house, career issues may be a factor, and, as the tenth rules one of our parents, it may also point to issues with that parent or authority figures in general. If Mercury is in the second, money problems may be a factor, or, in the seventh, relationships. Also look at any planets in the sixth house as they will have a say in the genesis and nature of the illness. Jupiter shows excess, and liver and blood conditions; Saturn, responsibility, and the musculoskeletal system. Again, this is a test of radicality. A disease shown by Virgo in the sixth will generally not be a hot illness, but a cold, dry condition (Virgo is melancholic) with a strong nervous component. (Remember, Virgo is ruled by Mercury the planet of the mind.) If there is more than one planet in the sixth house, the astrologer uses their craft to determine which of the planets has the most impact. Again, look back at the parts of the body the planets rule and their nature.

As you take your case history, look to the planets and signs and see what is flagged up. This is where the skill of the astrologer comes in; they will sift through the symbols to find the correct interpretation. This is no different from the herbalist who will sort and prioritize symptoms when taking a case history, and make a diagnosis through weighing up their relative importance, and then judge which of the hundreds of herbs available will be the most appropriate.

The practitioner

This is shown by the sign on the seventh house, the planet ruling the seventh house, and any planets in the seventh house. This is important information to consider before you meet the patient. This shows who your client wishes to see. Obviously, you cannot change your character, but it will indicate if they wish for sympathy, shown by the Moon, encouragement shown by a Fire sign, hope shown by Jupiter, or a strict regime, shown by Saturn. I feel this is vital information as it puts the patient at the centre of the consultation and it gives the practitioner insight into how to proceed with the consultation. It prevents a "factory line" approach to clients for, in any given day, you will express different sides to your nature according to necessity. It also avoids irritating your clients; if they want you to be upbeat, a saturnine approach with a fierce exclusion diet will not go down well. Some clients want to be told what to do, some want their ideas to be supported, some want all the news, good and bad, others just want a hopeful, positive message. Look to the seventh house and its ruler for clues.

Again, it is useful to look back and see how clients whose treatment was successful differed from those who did not return after a first appointment. It may be that their decumbiture shows they were looking for something you did not give them, particularly if, for example, you dislike rules and strict regimes and so rarely use them, while the patient wanted the safety and comfort of a saturnine experience.

The medicine

The tenth house and its ruler and any planets in the tenth house will show the medicine that the client needs. Here, knowledge of the planetary rulers of herbs comes in, but also herbal skill and choice-making.

The tenth shows the medicine, but Culpeper also has rules about prescribing:

> Fortify the body with herbs of the nature of the lord of the ascendant, 'tis no matter whether he be a fortune or an infortune in this case.
>
> Let your medicine be something antipathetical to the lord of the sixth.
>
> Let your medicine be something of the sign ascending.
>
> If the lord of the tenth be strong, make use of his medicines.
>
> If this cannot well be, make use of medicines of the light of time (Sun in a day time chart, Moon in a night time chart).
>
> Be sure to always fortify the grieved part of the body by sympathetical remedies.
>
> Regard the heart, keep that upon the wheels, because the Sun is the fountain of life.(Culpeper, 1806, p. 301.)

This allows for six or seven herbs in a prescription, although some herbs will double up in their actions. For example, if the chart shows Leo rising then a solar herb may also be a heart herb or, if you use a remedy for the "grieved part of the body", it may also be lord of the sixth or tenth house. Also, herbs may be given as tinctures, teas, or powders to increase the variety of herbs given.

This prescription sounds more complicated than it is in practice. Working with both the decumbiture and a case history, the practitioner will have an idea of where they are going with diagnosis and treatment. The decumbiture narrows down the possible remedies to pick. If, for example, you are looking for a remedy to support the liver, there are many: Dandelion and Milk Thistle, herbs of Jupiter, Wormwood and Holy Thistle, herbs of Mars, Marigold, herb of the Sun; what the decumbiture will do is narrow your choice down. To follow this example, if a liver remedy is required chose one that is a herb of Jupiter, in sympathy with the condition, or a herb of Mars in antipathy to what is showing as the sixth house ruler. I will add a few case histories where you can see the practice in action.

Sympathy and antipathy

This is a very important principle in any holistic practice, and also pivotal for decumbiture. Treating in sympathy is like the Hippocratic *vis medicatrix naturae*, and uses the force, wisdom, and intelligence of nature to cure the disease. For example, herbs of Venus are used to treat gynaecological conditions by sympathy, as Venus rules the reproductive system, similarly, Saturnine herbs are useful for dry skin conditions like psoriasis, because Saturn rules the skin and dryness in general. As Culpeper recommends:, "as the cause, so is the cure" (Culpeper, 1798, unnumbered page).

However, sometimes the symptoms are so severe that antipathetical remedies are called for, for example: heavy bleeding (a hot and moist condition) can be treated by cold and dry remedies, such as Shepherd's Purse, a herb of Saturn (Brooke, 2018, p. 185). The beauty of a herbal prescription is that, as outlined above, sympathetical remedies can be mixed with antipathetical. In haemorrhage, a cold, dry remedy can be used for the immediate alleviation of symptoms, while a warm, moist, sanguine remedy (the sanguine humour being concerned with blood) can be used to treat the underlying cause of the heavy bleeding. A heart remedy can be given both for hope and courage, and for the physical heart.

The end of the matter

The fourth house, the planet ruling the cusp of the fourth, and any planets in the fourth house will show how the matter ends. Clearly, Jupiter ruling or situated in the fourth house will be a good omen, while Saturn there is an indication that the disease will take a long time or never be cured. Pluto might show the client disappears, or that there will be a crisis, and the Moon suggests that things get better but return, wax and wane.

Eighth house

The eighth house is traditionally the house of death and surgery. Clearly predicting death is not one of the modern astrologer's skills and, as mortality is lower than it was in Culpeper's day, the practitioner is rare who tells a patient to put their affairs in order, as death is expected imminently. Operations, on the other hand, are all too common and the decumbiture will give insight into prognoses for the procedure and whether to delay elective surgery, or what the outcome of the surgery might be. Traditionally, any malefic in the eighth house, Saturn or Mars, is an evil omen, but as Mars rules surgery its presence there can be a good sign, depending on how Mars is placed. After all, if one has to have surgery, a skilled surgeon is most desirable.

Twelfth house

In traditional astrology, the twelfth house is the house of witchcraft and secret enemies. Sickness due to witchcraft was readily diagnosed in Culpeper's day, especially diseases which suddenly appeared and were resistant to treatment. A less common diagnosis now, the twelfth house has been renamed the house of self-undoing and this fits well with modern beliefs about sickness and health. Jupiter in the twelfth house of a decumbiture, or Venus, suggests self-indulgence might be a factor in the genesis of the illness. Venus loves sweet things, and sugar is known to cause many ailments from diabetes, to heart attacks, cancer, and thrush. Jupiter governs excesses; this may include over-eating, or excessive under-eating (I have seen this in the charts of anorexics), or any excessive activity: drinking, eating meat, exercising, and over-working come to mind. The twelfth is also the house of confinement; prisons are an obvious indication, but also hospitals, nursing homes, asylums, retreat centres, ashrams, and health farms. Planets in the twelfth may show a stay in hospital or the need to retreat and recuperate from whatever life-conditions have contributed to the sickness.

The other houses

Although not used in diagnosis or treatment plans, a quick look at the other houses of the decumbiture may give clues as to the genesis of the illness and possible remedial actions.

Seventh house

The seventh house rules marriage, friendships, and open enemies, of which marriage is the most germane. Unhappy relationships over the long-term wear down the spirit and can cause depression and physical symptoms of stress and unhappiness, which translate into bodily illness. These range from gut problems, to arthritis and heart disease, to reproductive issues and skin conditions. A tutor of mine once recommended, although not to the patient herself, that she needed a "husband-ectomy". Unhappy relationships are the cause of much misery and illness, but your discretion and common sense will determine how you use this information. Herbs can build up the heart, as Culpeper suggests, and give the person the courage to leave an unbearable situation.

Fifth house

The fifth house rules lovers and children. Clearly, lovers bring another spectrum of issues that may be translated into physical illness. Heart remedies will also be helpful here. The issue of children, childlessness, and empty-nesters will also be emphasized in the fifth house and can be addressed with sympathy and tact. If the client is coming about fertility problems, I would expect to see planets in the fifth house and I would look at the house and the planet ruling the fifth, and its condition, for clues about fertility and likely conception. Fertile planets are the Moon, Venus, and sometimes Jupiter and the Sun; fertile signs are the Water signs, especially Cancer and Pisces, and the Earth sign, Taurus. Infertile planets are Saturn and Mars; infertile signs are Capricorn, Aries, and Aquarius. However, the condition of the Moon in the decumbiture has a bigger say in whether conception will occur; consider its sign and house and next aspect.

Second house

The second house concerns money. Money troubles can be a real issue in stress-related diseases. There is not much a practitioner can do about this issue except perhaps to start the conversation. However, meanness is not simply about available wealth, it may relate to the way a person treats themselves. There may be a place for the practitioner to talk about self- care, cutting back on self-criticism, and relaxing strict rules, austere exclusion diets, or exercise regimes. Venus and the sign of Taurus traditionally rule money, while Mars and Scorpio rule debt, other people's money, and inherited wealth.

Third, ninth, and eleventh houses

These rule siblings (third), higher education, religion[7] and long-distance travel (ninth), and communities and groups in general (eleventh). Sometimes issues around these themes arise if the Moon or the significator

---

[7]Arguably, spirituality is more germane to the ninth house and religion to the tenth, because religion is often concerned with parent-like control and the public status of the member of the religion. Religion, especially if it is a particularly severe and punitive sort, can of course cause anxiety and depression. Certain religions chose herbal remedies rather than allopathic medicine, but, in my experience, astrology is anathema to them. The decumbiture method, of course, does not need to be overt, and can be used discretely in such cases with great success.

for either the disease or the client is in one of these houses, but, again, there is not much that can be done with them except to introduce these subjects into the consultation.

The Moon

By far the most important planet in the decumbiture is the Moon. The Moon takes approximately twenty-eight days to go through each sign of the zodiac, therefore, within a lunar month the Moon will touch each planet in a decumbiture. By so doing it will highlight the nature and property of that planet. Because of its changeable nature, the aspects the Moon makes to planets in the decumbiture and in the sky will reveal how the disease will progress. After one lunar month, the disease is said to no longer be acute and the movement of the Sun will be used to make timing judgements.

The Moon is co-significator of the disease and sometimes the patient. Look to the Moon when the planet ruling the disease (sixth house cusp) and the patient (ascendant) are the same; for example, when Aries rules the sixth house and Scorpio rules the ascendant (both are ruled by Mars). In such a case, look to the Moon to give further information.

The planet the Moon separates from, its house and condition, will show you the cause of the sickness and the state of the sick. Consider the planets the Moon applies to, their condition, benevolent and malevolent, moveable or fixed, hot, cold, dry, or moist, and what parts a planet governs, what diseases it owns, whether in an angle, and, especially, the house it is in and what part of the body it rules (Culpeper, 1651a, p. 73).

Timing measures, acute and chronic conditions

Another excellent way to use the decumbiture is for highlighting the optimal times for treatment. Acute disease is said to last one lunar month; that is, from the time the decumbiture was drawn to the same time one month later, when the Moon reaches the same degree and minute of the sign it was in, having travelled all around the chart. As discussed above, the Moon travels through all the planets in the decumbiture in the course of a lunar month. It will go over the planet representing the sick person and the planet(s) representing the sickness.

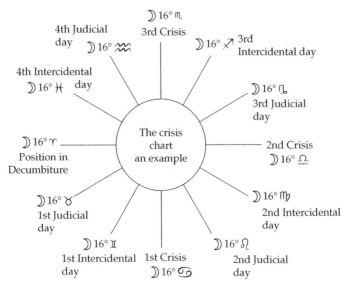

Figure 2. A crisis chart.

A crisis chart is drawn up (see Figure 2) with the sign and degree of the Moon in the decumbiture in the place of the ascendant. Within the lunar cycle there will be three crisis days. The first crisis is approximately seven days after the decumbiture was cast, where the Moon is square the decumbiture Moon. For example, if the decumbiture Moon is at 16° Aries, the first crisis will be when the Moon reaches 16° Cancer. The second crisis will be seven days later (or fourteen days after the decumbiture) when the Moon is at 16° Libra in our example. The third crisis will be when the Moon is at 16° Capricorn, twenty-one days after the decumbiture, and the final crisis when the Moon is back in the same position as in the decumbiture, 16° Aries, approximately one month later.

On crisis days there may be an exacerbation of symptoms. Planets involved should show the nature of the crisis. This is helpful to practitioners to weather the progress of the client, because it is rare that healing takes a straight road.

Especially helpful when planning appointments or treatments are the judicial days. These occur when the moon is making favourable aspects to the Moon in the decumbiture. So, in our example, the first judicial day is when the Moon is at 16° Taurus, the second when he Moon reaches 16° Leo (making a helpful trine aspect), the third judicial day is about sixteen days after the decumbiture when the Moon is in 16° Scorpio and the final judicial day is around twenty-three days after the decumbiture when the Moon is in 16° Aquarius. These are days to do any hands-on treatments, or to schedule appointments for an encouraging conversation and to adjust the medicine. Between the judicial days and the crisis days are the intercidental days, which are also favourable for treatments and conversation.

This may seem to be very complicated, but drawing the chart is straightforward and it gives a useful reminder for when to schedule appointments and treatments and what to bear in mind should there be a crisis in the treatment. A skilled practitioner can look at the planets involved in the crisis days and speak the language of those planets to reassure a worried patient.

Here are two simple decumbiture charts showing the method.

Tonsillitis

A contacted me saying she had been become ill with tonsillitis and fever with earache after having a Swedish massage. I drew up the chart (see Figure 3, below).

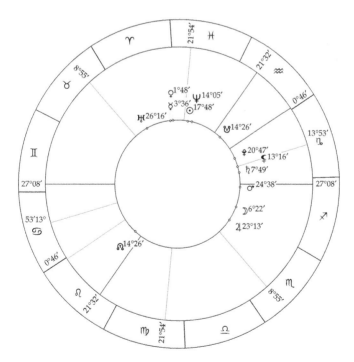

Figure 3. Decumbiture chart, example 1. 8 March, 2018, 10:32 hrs.

The patient is shown by the first house, and the planet ruling it. Gemini is rising and Mercury (ruler of Gemini) is in Aries in the eleventh house. The sickness is shown by the sign ruling the sixth house, the planet ruling this sign, and any planets in the sixth house. The illness is shown by Mars in Sagittarius in the sixth house (ruler of Scorpio). In the sixth house is Jupiter and the Moon in Sagittarius. I judged that the sickness was blood corrupted (Jupiter in Scorpio, Jupiter rules the blood, Scorpio can show corruption or poisoning, the Moon in Sagittarius echoes this theme). Sagittarius also shows over-heated fluids (Sagittarius is hot and moist) the ruler of the sickness, and over-heated Mars in Sagittarius again shows heat, fever, and corrupted blood.

Jupiter and Mars are in each other's signs; Jupiter rules Sagittarius, Mars rules Scorpio. Jupiter rules the seventh house of the physician and is placed in the sixth house. It could be argued that I, as physician, might be a cause of the illness. But I had not be treating her, so this could not be me. Perhaps the Jupiter shows the masseuse; remember that the illness came on after a massage. So, what did happen? Perhaps the massage overtaxed her liver (Jupiter) and released toxins (Scorpio) which overwhelmed her (Jupiter shows excess) and she became ill.

There is a planet in the seventh house, and this may show me the other practitioner. This is Saturn in Capricorn, which may show an older person (Saturn rules old age), and possibly an authority figure (Capricorn).

The medicine is shown by Aquarius on the tenth house cusp. Aquarius is co-ruled by Saturn and Uranus. This shows the physician that Saturn will be part of the client's healing. Furthermore Uranus is another part of the medicine, and Uranus rules astrology, which will be another part of the healing process.

The prescription I gave followed some of Culpeper's guidelines.

So, there is a theme of heat, poisoning, the liver, and a choleric-sanguine condition. Mars also rules the sign that Mercury is in (Aries). "Something of the nature of the ascendant", says Culpeper, in this case Mercury, so I prescribed White Horehound. "Something of the nature of the illness"; I gave Nettle, which is a herb of Mars, and Dandelion root and Meadowsweet, both herbs of Jupiter, because it is in the sixth house. And finally a remedy antipathetical to the sickness, a cooling remedy, Cleavers, ruled by the Moon.

The prescription:

Equal parts: Nettle
                Dandelion Root
                Meadowsweet
                White Horehound
                Cleavers. 10 drops of tincture every hour until symptoms go.

I also suggested that she stop worrying and thinking (I knew she was studying for a master's degree and was writing up her thesis) and give her mind a rest. Jupiter and Sagittarius rule higher education. She was also shown as the Mercury in Aries; again, thinking, and maybe speed, and the Moon was just separating from a trine (a good aspect) from the Mercury, which reinforced the theme of education (Moon in Sagittarius). She admitted that "communication and writing are great challenges of mine", which echoes the themes of the chart.

I saw her a few days later. She said she had taken the medicine, and the same day had had an acupuncture treatment (I give Uranus, ruler of the tenth, to acupuncture) and both treatments had resulted in the symptoms disappearing that same day. It could be argued it was the acupuncture, but I feel it was all three moves: the medicine and astrology, the acupuncture, and finally the acknowledgement that she needed silence and rest from her mental exertions.

Her feedback was: "I was so impressed by the accuracy of the astrological reading and the speed of recovery. Swollen tonsils, difficulty and painful swallowing, piercing left ear-ache, voice lost, exhaustion, joint pain in fingers, wrist, knees, and ankle. Last memorable experience of something similar was aged sixteen, on the right ear. Forty-five minutes after taking tincture mix recommended by you, every ten minutes, voice was regained, able to swallow and eat without pain. Close to a miracle!"

Period

A young woman came with amenorrhoea and digestive problems. She had recovered from an eating disorder but had not had a period for eleven years. She also suffered from a lot of digestive discomfort, bloating, wind, and constipation. Otherwise her health was fair, a bit of low energy, but B12 vitamins had helped with that.

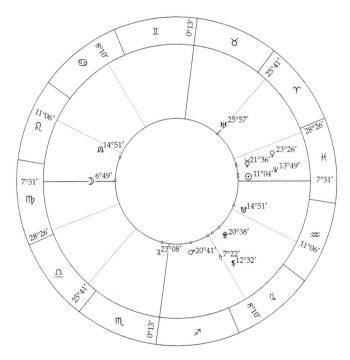

Figure 4. Decumbiture chart, example 2. 1 March, 2018. 17:15 hrs

The ascendant shows the Moon rising in Virgo. It showed the client as being of a melancholic disposition (Virgo, a melancholic Earth sign) who was also studying herbalism, as Virgo shows medicine and healing. The Moon is applying to the full Moon, but a trine to Saturn on the cusp of the fifth house comes first. Saturn also co-rules the sixth house of sickness with Uranus in the ninth house of astrology. Saturn again shows a melancholic condition. The other significator of the client is Mercury (a melancholy planet), ruler of the ascendant, mute in Pisces in the seventh house.

I prescribed Liquorice (a herb of Mercury) for the nature of the ascendant and its ruler. Liquorice is a great remedy for the gut, and is a demulcent, lubricating and softening, getting things moving. Motherwort (ruled by Venus) is "of the nature of the disease" (i.e., gynaecological, ruled by Venus). Melissa (ruled by Jupiter) is in antipathy to the melancholic illness; a fine gut remedy for wind and digestion, a gentle liver remedy, and a gynaecological tonic. Finally, Borage (also ruled by Jupiter), an adrenal trophorestorative for the stress of

worrying (Moon in Virgo), and also because it rules Pisces, the sign
Mercury was in. I also prescribed a tea of Mugwort (ruled by Venus)
to be taken 1–2 times a day. Mugwort is an emmenagogue and reproductive remedy.

I had a text two weeks later to say she had been taking the herbal tea
for ten days and the tincture for three days and had had her first period
for eleven years and was delighted.

Mary's red flower

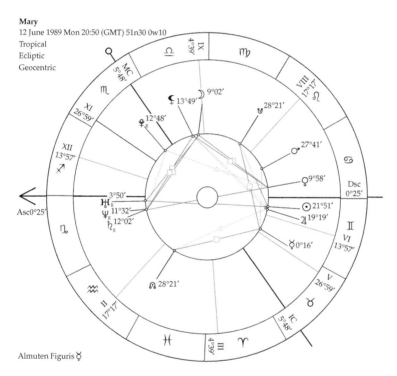

Figure 5. Decumbiture chart with timing, example 3. 12 June, 1989.
20:50 hrs.

A close friend and colleague called me in some distress. She had
had a slight bloody discharge and had gone to her GP. On examination
the doctor said there was a growth on her cervix and it was possibly
malignant. My friend was warned that this would mean an operation to remove the growth and a dilation and curettage, with possible

further investigatory surgery. Naturally she was very upset and called for my advice and support. I drew up a decumbiture chart for the time of the phone call and looked for either positive or negative signs.

The chart had Capricorn rising, so she was shown as the querent as Saturn. Saturn was in the first house of the chart and well-placed in Capricorn (Saturn is co-ruler of Capricorn). Lilly says the ruler of the ascendant should always physically describe the appearance of the patient and this should be the first test of a chart's radicality. Indeed, Mary had a saturnine/melancholic appearance: slim, dark, with thick, dark hair. Temperamentally, she also had a melancholic nature: intelligent, thoughtful, and prone to melancholy.

Saturn is strong in its own sign of Capricorn, but was retrograde and conjunct Neptune (which can be taken to be a negative influence; Neptune's nature is so opposite from Saturn's). From this I understood that her constitution was basically strong but had been weakened by its retrograde motion and a conjunction with Neptune. Neptune tends to "leak" energy and physically shows tiredness, vague feelings of illness and debility, as well as fearfulness.

The sickness is shown by Mercury, ruler of the sixth house, strong in its own sign of Gemini, in the fifth house, lately separating from a trine of the Moon. Mercury in the fifth suggests the cause of the illness relates to children, and M. was the mother of two under-fives. Perhaps it also shows a connection with childbirth trauma. I wondered if this related to the death of her first child as a newborn, or to the stresses and strains of coping with two pre-school children. Mercury is a melancholic planet and shows depression and nervous tension.

Besides studying the sixth house ruler, it is important to look at any planets in this house, as they give further clues as to the nature of the illness. In the sixth house are the Sun and Jupiter conjunct in Gemini. Both these planets are benefic and tend to bring good fortune to any matter. However, the Sun is ruler of the eighth house of death and surgery, which is not such a good sign. Furthermore, Jupiter rules the twelfth house of hospitals and self-undoing and is in detriment in Gemini. Although Jupiter brings good fortune, it is somewhat qualified. However, on balance I felt these were good-omened planets. The Sun and Jupiter also, to me, showed the physicality of the sickness: a growth (Jupiter) on the cervix (the glyph of the Sun ⊙ representing the physical appearance of the cervix, which is a doughnut shape with a small opening). So indeed, there was a growth, but my reading was that it would be benign and not malignant.

The Moon, co-significator of the question, was found in the ninth house in Libra. The Moon was about to make a square to Venus, which spoke to me of the nature of the illness (Venus representing the reproductive system, Cancer the mother). The mutual reception of the Moon and Venus (in each other's signs, as Venus rules Libra and the Moon rules Cancer) together with Venus's rulership of the fifth house of children further echoes the theme. A square is an aspect of stress and shows how her female body was in conflict, resulting in physical symptoms. The Moon then goes on to make an aspect to Saturn and Neptune by square. I saw this as indicating there would be anaesthetics (Neptune), affecting the tissues of the body (Saturn). The Moon later moves to a trine to the Sun/Jupiter easing up the threat from Saturn.

I felt the outcome would be favourable. I predicted a minor operation, but not a dilation and curettage, and that the tumour would be found to be a benign growth (Jupiter ruling growths and being benign), probably a polyp.

I saw that her constitution, shown by Saturn, needed building up, so I prescribed Comfrey and Horsetail, both herbs of Saturn, and also Dandelion root, a herb of Jupiter, to oppose the sickness (Jupiter opposes Mercury) and at the same time as a remedy to rebalance the author of the sickness, Mercury, I prescribed Valerian (ruled by Mercury).

As the practitioner I am shown as the ruler of the seventh house, which is Cancer and is ruled by the Moon. The Moon is in Libra in the ninth house of astrology, showing the physician is also an astrologer. My natal Moon is in Libra, although not at this degree, and so further demonstrates the chart was radical for my involvement. The Venus on the descendant also shows another physician. Because it is Venus in Cancer I felt it related to the gynaecologist (Venus rules the reproductive system). The Moon is applying to the square of Venus, which I felt suggested our two different approaches, which were at odds with one another (a square is an aspect of tension and difficulty). Venus is well-placed in Cancer and disposes my Moon in Libra (as Venus rules Libra) so, in the short term, I felt the gynaecologist's approach would prevail, and that Mary would follow her treatment. However, my Moon also disposes the Venus (as the Moon rules Cancer) so I believed my treatment, which would be a mixture of herbs, astrology, and comfort (the Moon), would also have a benign influence.

As discussed earlier, a decumbiture as the astrology of katarche shows a relationship unfolding between the questioner and the practitioner. It allows the questioner to move forward on the issue and seek a resolution or healing, or at least make an informed decision on what to do next. This decumbiture laid out clearly Mary's options. As a herbalist herself, Mary was against medical intervention. But she was afraid (Saturn/Neptune shows her fear and foreboding) that the condition might turn out to be malignant and that a simple operation could result in a cure, the benefic Sun and Jupiter in the sixth house of sickness bringing hope, and particularly as the Sun rules the eighth house of operations. Mary reasoned she could not take the risk (Saturn, her significator, is very risk averse) but had to break free from her strongly held beliefs (Saturn), and embody Uranus, the planet of splits and revolution, which was conjunct her Capricorn ascendant.

The decumbiture also gives the herbalist an opportunity to discover what kind of practitioner the patient requires and how they might best move forward on the case. The physician shown as the Moon in Libra (a dual sign) was weighing up (a very Libran activity) the two possibilities: herbal treatment, or orthodox medical treatment. Perhaps this was a heart versus head dilemma, the head being Libra (an Air sign, so rational and thoughtful), and the heart or emotion being the Moon. Being a dual sign, my judgement was to not choose one method or the other, but both. I suggested Mary should elect to have the exploratory operation, and at the same time take healing and restorative herbs to build up her strength and begin her recovery. I also felt, as a rational Libra, that my task was to remain cool-headed and detached (as Air signs are) because Mary was fearful and the other physician, showed by Venus in Cancer, was reacting emotionally (the Moon), as doctors sometimes do when they are sure the treatment they are recommending is correct.

What follows is another use for the decumbiture method: timing.

Timing

In decumbiture it is possible to follow a course of an illness and pick the optimum time for treatment and look out for possible crises and take remedial measures.

Acute illnesses

In decumbiture an illness is defined as acute if it has lasted less than one lunar month, around twenty-eight days. A crisis chart is cast which takes as its ascendant the degree and sign of the Moon in the decumbiture (see Figure 6, below). The first crisis day will be when the Moon has travelled from the decumbiture sign and degree to make a square or ninety-degree aspect. So, if the decumbiture Moon is at 10° Aries, the first crisis day/time will be when the Moon reaches 10° Cancer, about one week later. The Second crisis day will be when the Moon is opposite

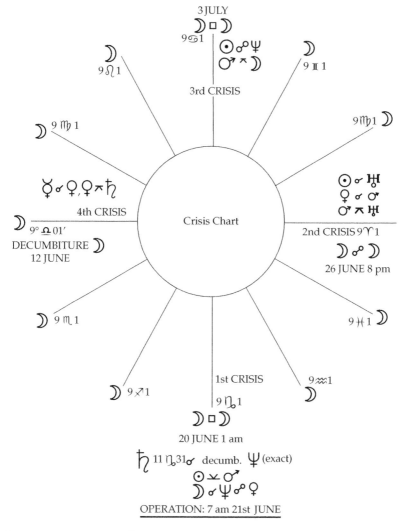

Figure 6. Mary's crisis chart.

the decumbiture Moon, in our example, 10° Libra, around fourteen days after the decumbiture. The third crisis day will be when the Moon is square the decumbiture Moon, or about three weeks after the decumbiture chart, in this case 10° Capricorn. Between the crisis days there are intercidental days, or beneficial days. In our example, they would be when the Moon is at 10° Taurus, Gemini, Leo, Virgo, Scorpio, Sagittarius, Aquarius, and Pisces. These would be good days to do a treatment or schedule a visit. On the crisis days, look at the planets and any aspects they make to get a sense of what form the crisis may take. I know this all sounds very complicated, but once you have done it a few times it makes sense.

Chronic illness

Once the Moon has arrived back at the original position in the decumbiture, in around twenty-nine days, the illness has become chronic. Then you take the degree and sign of the Sun in the decumbiture and you plot a chart for a year, the time it takes for the Sun to come back to its original position in the decumbiture. The crisis days will be every three months and the intercidental days every month, when the Sun is at the same degree as it was in the decumbiture, i.e. 10° Taurus, Gemini, Cancer, etc., in our example chart.

So, back to Mary

I drew up a crisis chart using the Moon to see what the likely outcome would be. The first crisis came in the early hours of the morning, on Tuesday 20 June. Saturn was retrograding back onto the decumbiture Neptune, and the Sun made a semi-sextile to the decumbiture Mars. This spoke to me of anaesthetics and possibly the knife (as Mars rules sharp objects). In the sky, the Moon was also conjunct Neptune and opposite Venus, which further pointed to an operation involving female organs.

At the second crisis, the Sun was opposite the decumbiture Uranus, Venus widely conjunct the decumbiture Mars, and Mars was inconjunct the decumbiture Uranus (an inconjunct is an aspect of sickness). My feeling about this second crisis was that there would be more local surgery (Mars) perhaps involving laser treatment (Uranus, which rules technology) but that the Sun/Jupiter conjunction in the decumbiture showed a good outcome.

At the third crisis the Sun was opposite the decumbiture Neptune, and Mars was widely sextile the Moon. I took this to mean possible weakness (Neptune) and slight fever (Mars). The forth crisis showed Mercury conjunct the decumbiture Venus (Mercury ruling the illness, Venus showing the gynaecologist), so the illness comes to the physician, and Venus inconjunct the decumbiture Saturn. My feeling was that this would be the final crisis and there would be a resolution and reconciling of Mercury, the sickness.

A few days later I had a call from Mary to say she had seen the consultant at the hospital. She was reassured that there was a ninety-nine per cent probability that the growth was benign. (Remember the benefic Sun/ Jupiter in the house of sickness.) Furthermore, a simple local operation (Mars) was needed but no dilation and curettage, nor would she have to stay overnight in hospital and be away from her eleven-month old child.

Mary's operation

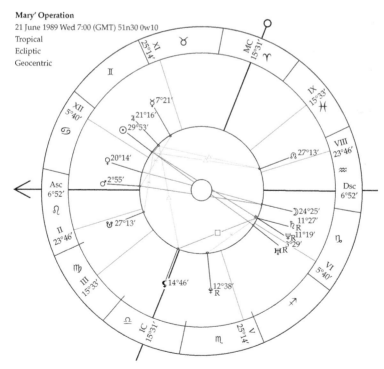

Figure 7. Chart for Mary's operation. 21 June, 1989, 0730 hrs.

The operation was set for 21 June at 7am GMT. We talked about the timing differences of the first crisis when I had predicted the operation would take place and the anaesthetic. On that first crisis the Moon was in Capricorn, applying to the Saturn of the decumbiture, and Mary's healing journey was beginning, the Moon applying to Neptune showing an anaesthetic. Mary had looked at the polyp and it resembled a red flower growing under the surface of the cervix. The consultant thought it might have been due to childbirth trauma. (Mercury, significator of the sickness, is found in the fifth house of children in the decumbiture.)

I also looked up in the ephemeris to see when Saturn, significator of Mary would stop being retrograde (go direct), and saw it was on 11 September. I predicted that by then she would be fully recovered, especially as, on that same day, Mercury, author of the illness, would go retrograde—back off and weaken, in other words.

Mary felt that this event had been a warning to her against wearing herself out with hard work and looking after her children (Saturn). I also wondered if her high ideals about mothering (Neptune) might be setting her an impossible task. Neptune conjunct Saturn in the decumbiture, showed how fear and unrealistic expectations, all Neptunian problems, were pressing down on her already tired and retrograde Saturn. The decumbiture Saturn mirrored Mary's natal Saturn in Libra on the ascendant; both her strength to overcome a setback (Saturn) and her need for balance (Libra).

I then drew up a chart for the time of the operation. The chart shows Mary as the Sun in Gemini (ruling the ascendant) separating from Jupiter, indicating that she was separating herself from her growth (Jupiter). A dignified Mars in Leo conjunct the ascendant shows the surgery supports the querent. The sickness is shown by the ruler of the sixth, a retrograde Saturn in the sixth with Neptune indicating an anaesthetic. Interestingly, these significators are the reverse of the significators of the decumbiture. Now Saturn shows the sickness and the Sun the patient. The Moon, as universal co-significator of the chart, is badly placed in Capricorn in the sixth house and makes no major aspects before it leaves Capricorn. As mentioned previously, void of course Moons signify nothing will come of the matter, which could mean the surgery will not take place, or, as I judged, it will happen, but no further treatment will be needed.

Surgery is shown by the ruler of the eighth house, Saturn or Uranus, which co-rules Aquarius. Interestingly, Uranus is in the fifth house while Saturn is in the sixth, so there is a choice of interpretations here. Taking Saturn, the traditional ruler of Aquarius, it pushes the ruler of the twelfth, the Moon, which is in his sign of Capricorn. Traditionally the ruler of the eighth house of surgery (and death) in the sixth house is ill-omened, and clearly there are risks with any surgery. But it is not the significator of Mary but of her illness, so I take it to mean the illness is weakening its hold on Mary and does not have enough strength to better the querent, the Sun in Jupiter.

The end of the matter is shown by the fourth house cusp, Venus well-placed in Cancer in the twelfth house of hospital. The twelfth house is traditionally an unlucky house, sometimes called the house of self-undoing and self-sacrifice. I feel this relates to Mary's self-sacrifice caring for her children, shown by a motherly Venus in Cancer. The Moon is separating from an opposition to Venus, showing again that her sickness is leaving.

One year after the operation, there had been no further symptoms and no other treatment was required. Both physicians had been successful, the surgeon and the herbalist, and the patient had taken on board changes needed in her life to prevent her falling ill again.

The treatment

From a herbalist's perspective, the remedies I gave would not be those which automatically spring to mind when contemplating treating such a condition. It was a disease of the reproductive system, yet I prescribed no gynaecological herbs; instead I prescribed herbs that would traditionally have been used for the musculoskeletal system, Comfrey and Horsetail. My rationale was not to treat the condition so much as to strengthen the vital spirit or constitution of the patient and allow nature (*vis medicatrix naturae*) to do the healing. Constitutionally, as we discussed, Mary was melancholic, but her ruling planet, shown in the decumbiture as Saturn was retrograde. Mary, by nature, was strong (Saturn rules Capricorn) but momentarily debilitated (retrograde). For that reason, I felt her natural vital spirit, had the innate strength to fight the disease, but needed some help as it was momentarily weakened through overwork and too much responsibility (Saturn). Following the Hippocratic dictum, if the nature of the patient is momentarily weakened, but fundamentally strong, allow nature to do its job of healing by holistically treating them with remedies which make them strong enough to heal themselves. And this is what happened. There was no recurrence of the illness.

This chart shows how helpful decumbiture can be in *katarche*, by entering into the issue with the patient and providing moral support, answers to questions, and remedies that strengthen the constitution of the patient; a real holistic practice.

The next chart illustrates the method perfectly. This was the first timing chart I had used to give a specific treatment.

The case of the missing gallstones

A man came to see me who had been referred by a friend of mine who felt herbal treatment might be helpful in his condition. Some weeks previously the man had a frightening attack of what turned out to be pancreatitis, inflammation of the pancreas. It transpired that this had been caused by gallstones distending his gallbladder, causing it to swell and to put pressure on his pancreas. He was in a distressed condition and wanted to know if I could help.

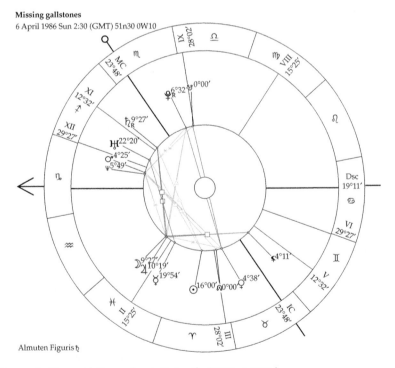

Figure 8. Decumbiture chart. 6 April, 1986. 1430 hrs.

Because he was able to exactly locate the time his illness began, I drew up a decumbiture for that time: 2.30pm on 6 April, 1986.

In the decumbiture the sick man is shown by the ruler of the ascendant, Saturn in Sagittarius, the cold, dry nature of Saturn at odds with the warmth and moisture of Jupiter. Saturn found in the tenth house of career suggests that the work life of the sick man may have had an effect on his health. The illness is shown by the planet ruling the cusp of the sixth house, the Moon in Pisces. The illness could then be described as having the nature of the Moon in Pisces, namely phlegmatic, cold, and wet. The illness may have been caused by an excess of fishy things, Pisces ruling the sea; it transpired that in the past he had eaten large quantities of tuna fish. Being wet and cold, Pisces can also be said to rule some types of alcohol. The man revealed that in the past he had been drinking two to four bottles of wine per week. Cancer ruling the sixth house points to the digestive system and the action of the stomach in particular, which leads us to expect the illness to be of digestive origin. The sick man was of an anxious disposition who admitted to worrying about things in general.

During the week leading up to the attack he suffered from stomach ache (Cancer, ruling the stomach) and had been passing yellow urine (Mars and Choler, yellow shows heat), which is represented by the Moon separating from Mars/Neptune conjunction. There was also stabbing pain caused by the gallbladder (Mars rules the gallbladder), together with a vague feeling of unease, which I took to be Neptune.

On the evening of the fifth he ate a rich meal of cauliflower cheese (Venus, in Taurus, likes rich food) and drank a bottle of wine (Moon in Pisces). At 2.30am the next morning he woke and was violently sick, which might have been triggered by the Moon trine Pluto in Scorpio (expelling poisons in a violent, explosive way). The Moon rules the expulsive faculty in the body, and Pluto in Scorpio possibly represents poisoned blood.

The next morning, he went to his doctor, also represented by the Moon, ruler of the seventh house cusp. The doctor sent him immediately to hospital; Saturn rules the ascendant and the twelfth house, representing hospitals. He was jaundiced in the left eye (the Moon rules the left eye in men). Jaundice, a liver disease, is ruled by Jupiter, the Moon applied to the conjunction of Jupiter. The treatment recommended was to fast for two days, and he was put on a saline drip (sea water, Pisces; also Water, the Moon, and salt-Saturn). The Moon was square Saturn. On the eighth he underwent blood tests, the Moon now in Aries in the first lunar cycle; Mars the ruler of red blood cells; and the Moon the ruler of bodily fluids. As a result of these tests they diagnosed acute pancreatitis and said the only possible treatment was surgery, shown by the Moon conjunction of Mercury, ruling the eighth house of surgery.

Because the operation did not have to happen immediately, he was able to negotiate with the doctors for time to consider the options. He left hospital soon afterwards and went to see his acupuncturist, who had been treating him for several years. The acupuncturist referred him onto me for herbal treatment. He was very reluctant to have the operation, which meant the removal of his gallbladder, wanting to explore all other options before taking this drastic step.

It was a difficult decision as the surgeon had stated that there were no other options open to him and that, if he delayed the operation for too long, he might put himself at greater risk, causing permanent damage to his pancreas. Such damage would be irreversible and could have serious consequences for his future health and wellbeing.

His first visit to me was on 14 May, by which time we were in the second month of his illness. In the decumbiture the physician is shown by the Moon in Pisces, a dual sign. My understanding was that for the first month the Moon represented the medical profession, and for the second month it represented my treatment. The Moon ruling both the sixth and seventh house cusps might show that the physician would increase the illness and it could be argued that the first physician, the medical profession, did offer that possibility by their drastic suggestion for treatment. Being a woman, I might represent a lunar influence and might work more in time with the Moon's cycles. Alternatively, I could be seen as an authority figure by the tenth house cusp, being the one who knows rather than the one who relates. I would then be seen as Mars, which has synastry with my own natal Mars. Yet Mars, representing the knife and surgery, could be seen as the medical profession. It was an ill-omened Mars as it was found in the twelfth house, indicating the physician compounding the self-undoing of the patient. It might represent the authority of the medical profession aiming to hospitalise him and cut his gallbladder (Mars). Pluto, as the co-ruler of the tenth, felt more appropriate for me as physician. I was aiming to bring to the surface hidden poisons that had collected in his system and expel them in an explosive way, all very Plutonian actions.

Pluto in the decumbiture was exactly my natal sixth house Saturn, ruler of my tenth house of career. Here, the Pluto can be read as my work being to challenge the authority of the medical profession.

To see the end of the illness I located the planet ruling the fourth house, Venus, which was also lady of the ninth house of astrology and opposing Pluto, significator of authority. This seemed to be an auspicious sign, that a cure would be effected with herbs, in the hands of a woman, reflecting my own natal Venus in Taurus rising.

Culpeper's rules for treatment are as follows:

"[C]onsider who is the author or cause of it [the disease] ... consider what planet governs that" (Culpeper, 1806, p. 301). Here the disease is shown by the Moon.

"[C]onsider whether it be caused by sympathy or antipathy of the planet" (Culpeper, 1806, p. 301). Coldness had made the bile solid and formed it into a stone, thus the disease is caused by sympathy, the Moon being a cold planet.

"Consider whether the planet afflicted do govern the part afflicted" (Culpeper, 1806, p. 301). The Moon does not govern the gallbladder, Mars does, but she does rule the digestive system, and so has some say over the liver and gallbladder. The Moon is antipathetical in nature to Mars, who is hot and dry. As Culpeper wrote: "as is the disease, so is the cure" (Culpeper, 1806, p. 301). I decided to use warm herbs, antipathetical to the nature of the Moon. This is, in a sense, working against nature, but I needed to move boldly to ease the stones from his gallbladder and to prepare him for the more drastic Mars cure that I had in mind. Culpeper says: "if by antipathy, then apply those medicines proper to the place affected, and governed by the afflicted parts" (Culpeper, 1806, p. 301). Jupiter rules the liver and opposes Saturn and the Moon, being warm and moist. The Sun opposes, being warm and dry. The Sun rules the vital spirit, which is needed in any acute illness, and after shock, to sustain and support life. I gave him the following herbs:

Dandelion root: a Jupiter herb, a remedy for the liver and gallbladder, helping to dissolve stones and wash them away by increasing the flow of bile from the liver.

Meadowsweet: which I give to Jupiter (Culpeper gives it to Venus). It is a general tonic and healer for the digestive system, and reduces the level of acid in the body.

Agrimony: ruled by Jupiter and astringent, which strengthens, cleanses, and tonifies the liver and the whole digestive system.

Marigold: another Sun remedy for both the liver and stomach, which strengthens, builds, and heals the tissues, and stimulates the digestive secretions.

I then set up a crisis chart using the Moon from the decumbiture chart for when he fell ill (see Figure 9, below). I used the lunar chart as I reasoned that the first lunar cycle represented his treatment with the doctors, and the second one would show the progress of his treatment with me. Although this is not traditional, because usually after the first lunar cycle timing measures are done with the movement of the Sun, it can be argued that this move is reflected by the Moon being in a dual sign (Pisces, the two fishes swimming in opposite directions) and the client having two physicians.

He first saw me on the fourteenth and took my medicine for four days. Then, as if on cue, on the eighteenth, when the Moon was opposite the decumbiture moon and square Saturn, he had another attack, less acute than the first, following a rich meal. The Moon was applying opposite to Jupiter and Mercury. So, the Moon was in hard aspect (square) to a malefic Saturn, which showed not only the sick man (the ascendant) but also the twelfth house of self-undoing. His over-indulgence had been

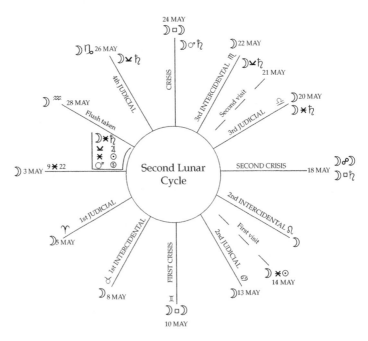

Figure 9. Crisis chart.

too much for his system and it had sent warning signals of pain to tell
him to stop. The Moon then moved on to the opposition of Jupiter, and
finally to oppose Mercury, which was ruler of the eighth house of death.
This was an ill-omened attack, which, appearing at the moment of the
second crisis proved the radicality of the crisis chart.

This was especially useful as I planned to give him a liver flush and
wanted to use my astrology to find the most auspicious time to start this
treatment. His next visit was 21 May, and we discussed the pros and
cons of the liver flush, the possible side effects and hoped-for results.
My overall feeling was that his illness was a healing crisis, or the surfac-
ing of an old problem (Mars in the twelfth) which, once resolved, would
not recur as his lifestyle had changed to such a degree I felt sure the
stones would not re-form.

The best days for treatment are judicial or intercidental days in the
crisis chart.

The next judicial day was 26 May. Here, the Moon would be in
Capricorn in detriment, semi-sextile Saturn, with Saturn disposing the
Moon. As well as the involvement with Saturn, the greater malefic,
and also a significator of stones (cold, dry action) I judged this was not
auspicious as the Moon would be in the twelfth house of the decumbiture separating from Mars, another malefic.

The next possible date was when the Moon was in Aquarius in
the first house of the decumbiture applying to the sextile of Saturn
(a helpful aspect) and the Moon was conjunct the part of sickness.[8] I felt
the best time to overcome the sickness was when the Moon was over the
part of sickness and Saturn, as the man disposited it.[9] After the Moon's
conjunction with the part of sickness, she goes on to make a sextile
(helpful) aspect to the Sun, which is strong in Aries, bringing hope of
success (the Sun) and a new beginning (Aries) of restored good health.
A further helpful aspect, the Moon moves from a sextile of Saturn to a
semi-sextile of Jupiter, the greater benefic, and dispositor of Saturn in
Sagittarius. For all these reasons I decided that when the Moon was at
9'22" of Aquarius would be an auspicious time for him to begin the
liver flush.

---

[8]The part of sickness is one of the Arabic parts in astrology, the part of fortune being the
most commonly used. The part of sickness is calculated by ascendant + Mars – Saturn.
[9]A planet disposes another when the first planet rules the sign the second planet is in.
In this case, Saturn, ruler of Aquarius, disposes or overpowers or neutralises the part of
sickness in Aquarius.

The liver flush involves using olive oil (ruled by the Moon), olives (Jupiter), and lemon juice (the Sun). Jupiter rules the liver; Pisces, a phlegmatic sign, stimulates the expulsive faculty, as does the Moon. Jupiter would soften the stones (Saturn). The patient had to fast for a few hours and then drink a large quantity (Jupiter) of olive oil, alternating it with lemon juice. The lemon juice would partially dissolve the stones and the oil would wash them out of the body.

He contacted me the next day to say it had all gone as planned. He had experienced a few twinges of his liver but generally was feeling fine. As he was due to go away for a few weeks, I gave him some more of the same medicine to heal and cleanse his system with instructions to contact me if he had any problems.

I saw him next in August and he reported that everything was fine; there had been the odd twinge but no recurrence of the severe symptoms. I decided I would now work to strengthen his nature, shown by Saturn in Sagittarius, so I gave him a mixture of Dandelion root and Horsetail, a remedy of Saturn, which cleanses the blood via the kidneys and builds up the strength and stamina of the body, while healing any wounded tissue.

He was due to return to hospital in September and we arranged to meet after he had the results of his scan. He called with the news that no stones were found on the scan. The doctors were amazed and could not understand how this was possible. Single stones sometimes work themselves out, but there had been so many when he had his first scan it was thought impossible that they had all disappeared. He reported they couldn't get him out of the room quickly enough, and did not wish to hear his explanation for what had happened.

To complete the healing process, and for any residual inflammation to be cleared up, I gave him medicine for another few months, after which time he reported even the minor twinges had gone. He had no further problems.

This was the first decumbiture I did using the crisis chart, and I feel it was a gift to me, showing how astrology can be used for diagnosis and treatment.

Temperament

In this chapter we will look at how we can work practically with the four elements and the four temperaments. It may be, as Culpeper and Lilly suggest, that planets in the natal sixth house denote chronic ill-health in some people, but it is not written that they should do so. People are complex and multi-layered. What might be expressed as physical illness in one person may present other challenges or issues in another. The danger of predicting health from the birth chart is that it might become a self-fulfilling prophecy. Our minds are powerful, as spiritual seekers have always known. What we imagine to be has a habit of becoming what is, in the same way that what we draw to us are those things we fear the most, because energy follows thought. Of course, it is useful to look at the natal chart, particularly in clients we have trouble helping, but the natal chart should mirror the decumbiture, and is best used as a test of radicality.

That said, determining temperament takes us away from pathology and into health. As Rudolph Steiner discovered, knowing one's temperament allows you to build on your strengths while minimizing your weaknesses (Greenbaum, 2005, p. 58). The descriptions of the regimes for the temperaments (see Part One, above) is a good place to start. Diet, exercise, and emotional wellbeing perform a pivotal role in maintaining health and happiness, as well as understanding what has happened when things go awry.

I have therefore, not chosen charts of "sick" people to illustrate the method, but of influential people in the world of healing and astrology, people who were key in my learning journey in these arts. Their life experiences, and in some cases health issues, illustrate the challenges and opportunities for each temperament.

The temperament of a person is their inherent physical, emotional, mental, and spiritual nature, their state of perfect health. Working with temperaments, the calculation of which involves looking at the natal chart, gives a picture of health rather than disease and offers guidelines and insight into a person's strengths and vulnerabilities, rather than their predicted pathologies. The temperament can be a pure type: choleric, sanguine, melancholic, or phlegmatic; or, more commonly, a mixed type with two or sometimes three of the humours emphasized.

The calculation works on the elemental qualities of the planets and signs in the nativity, as well as the season of birth, the phase of the Moon, and time of birth.[1] Below are the tables needed for the calculation and some worked-through examples.[2]

A worked example: Deepak Chopra

Calculation:

1. Temperament of the season: Deepak was born in Libra season (row 1, column 3) so it scores 2 for melancholic.
2. Temperament of ascendant sign: he has Pisces on the ascendant, so it scores 2 for phlegmatic (row 4, column 4).
3. Temperament of the ascendant ruler: Jupiter rules Pisces and Jupiter is sanguine, score 1 (row 3 column 1).
4. Temperament of the almuten: this is Venus, and Venus is a phlegmatic planet, so score 1 for phlegmatic (row 3 column 4).

---

[1]Unfortunately, if the time of birth is unknown it will be impossible to calculate the temperament. However, close questioning and some intuitive listening may provide an answer as the characteristics of temperaments are fairly easy to spot.

[2]I have used an amalgam of Lilly, Culpeper, and Geisler Greenbaum's (2005) methods. I have loosely used Greenbaum's system, but have taken short cuts (or liberties) with the method.

Table 1. Scoring table to calculate the temperament

	Score	Sanguine	Choleric	Melancholic	Phlegmatic
Temperament of the season	2				
Temperament of ascendant sign	2				
Temperament of ascendant ruler	1				
Temperament of almuten	1				
Temperament of Moon sign	2				
Temperament of Moon phase	1				
Temperament of planet ruling Moon sign	1				
	Total				

Table 2. Key to find the temperament in a natal chart[1]

	Sanguine	Choleric	Melancholic	Phlegmatic
Temperament of the season	Spring (which covers the signs of Aries, Taurus, and Gemini)	Summer (signs of Cancer, Leo, and Virgo)	Autumn (signs of Libra, Scorpio, and Sagittarius)	Winter (signs of Capricorn, Aquarius, and Pisces)
Temperament of the elements	Air	Fire	Earth	Water
Temperament of the planets	Jupiter	Mars, Sun	Saturn, Mercury	Venus, Moon
Temperament of the signs	Gemini, Libra, Aquarius	Aries, Leo, Sagittarius	Taurus, Virgo, Capricorn	Cancer, Scorpio, Pisces
Temperament of the Moon's phase	New to first quarter	First quarter to full	Full to last quarter	Last quarter to new

[1]Many thanks to Moira Paton and Joanna Watters and the other participants of my Astrology and Herbs week in Lefkada for helping me to re-design the table to make it more user-friendly and understandable.

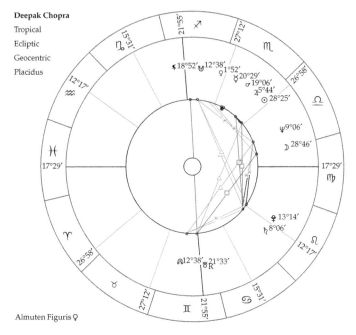

Figure 10. Temperament example 1. Deepak Chopra. 22 October 1946, 1545 hrs, New Delhi 28n36 77e12.

	Score	Sanguine	Choleric	Melancholic	Phlegmatic
Temperament of the season	2			2	
Temperament of ascendant sign	2				2
Temperament of ascendant ruler	1	1			
Temperament of almuten	1				1
Temperament of Moon sign	2			2	
Temperament of Moon phase	1				1
Temperament of planet ruling Moon sign	1			1	
	Total	1	0	5	4

5. Temperament of the Moon sign: the Moon sign is Virgo, which is a melancholic sign. Score 2 for melancholic (row 4 column 3).
6. Temperament of Moon phase: the Moon is applying to new, score 1 for phlegmatic (row 5 column 4).
7. Temperament of the planet ruling the Moon sign: the Moon is in Virgo, Virgo is ruled by Mercury, Mercury is a melancholic planet. Score 1 for melancholic (row 3 column 3).

So, Deepak is a melancholic phlegmatic, or 1-0-5-4 (the greater score comes first in the description). Melancholics are deep thinkers and secretly very ambitious. Chopra originally trained as an endocrinologist and currently is professor of public health at The University of California (status and public recognition are very important to power-seeking melancholics. He is one of the best-known practitioners of alternative medicine and meditation (phlegmatic). He was a disciple of Maharishi and offers free meditation courses to online participants worldwide (phlegmatic philanthropy). He is reputedly worth $80 million and has been accused to pandering to the rich. His courses can cost thousands of dollars (melancholic). He believes the mind affects the body, and in his model of the quantum body, thoughts can alter disease states and slow down ageing. (Melancholics like systems and patterns.) He is a hard-working melancholic, author of over eighty books including the New York Times bestseller, *The Seven Spiritual Laws of Success*, which, to my mind, encapsulates the practical, pragmatic melancholic with the mystical, spiritual phlegmatic.

Phlegmatic: Dr Elisabeth Kübler-Ross

Elisabeth Kübler-Ross is phlegmatic with some choleric, 6:3 points.

Kübler-Ross wrote the ground-breaking book *On Death and Dying* (1969) in which she outlined the five stages of dying: denial, isolation, anger, bargaining, depression and, finally, acceptance. She transformed the medical establishment's view of death. If any sign could be said to have an understanding of death it would be Pisces. But Uranus in the last degree of Pisces in the first house shows a revolution (Uranus) of how we think about death. Her compassionate Moon and Sun in Cancer (phlegmatic) show how she was impelled to do something about the way the dying were treated, as they were put in a side room and basically forgotten, as though there were something shameful about them. Kübler-Ross's Sun is conjunct the ruler of the eighth house

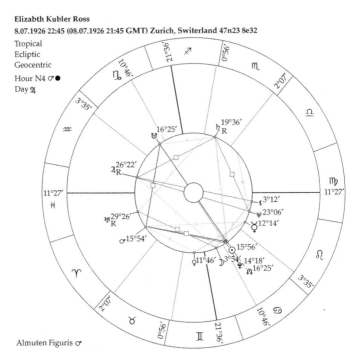

Elizabth Kubler Ross
8.07.1926 22:45 (08.07.1926 21:45 GMT) Zurich, Switerland 47n23 8e32

Tropical
Ecliptic
Geocentric
Hour N4 ♂●
Day ♃

Almuten Figuris ♂

Figure 11. Temperament example 2. Elisabeth Kübler-Ross. 08 July 1926, 21:45 hrs, Zurich 47n23 8e32.

	Score	Sanguine	Choleric	Melancholic	Phlegmatic
Temperament of the season	2		2		
Temperament of ascendant sign	2				2
Temperament of ascendant ruler	1	1			
Temperament of almuten	1		1		
Temperament of Moon sign	2				2
Moon phase	1				1
Temperament of Moon ruler	1				1
	Total	1	3	0	6

of death, Pluto, and is in the fifth house (phlegmatics will speak up for the marginalized and voiceless). Elisabeth Kübler-Ross confronted taboos (Pluto) about death (ruler of the eighth) in a creative way (Cancer, fifth house). The almuten of her chart is the fiery Mars in Aries, which is square her Sun-Pluto conjunction. She admitted she had an abrasive personality (Mars in Aries) but the gloriously fiery Mars would have just got things done. (Cholerics get the job done despite opposition; they fight for justice.) Mars is trine Mercury in Leo in the sixth house, which spread her message widely (Mercury in a Fire sign) and enlisted the help of influential people (Leo). The ruler of her ascendant and midheaven is Jupiter in the twelfth house in Aquarius. The twelfth house is the house of hospitals, where she worked. Denied a residency in paediatrics because she was pregnant, she took one in psychiatry from which her life's work developed. Kübler-Ross encouraged the hospice movement (phlegmatic compassion for the dying, hospices shown by the twelfth house). She believed euthanasia prevented people from completing their unfinished business (phlegmatic, spiritual perspective). The twelfth shows great compassion and a tuning into the zeitgeist; the world was ready to hear her message. The twelfth house is the house of the collective unconscious and psychic phenomena: Kübler-Ross discussed the phenomenon of near-death experiences, opening the dialogue in the mainstream. These are both phlegmatic areas of interest.

Ever one to confront taboos, compassion insisted she started a hospice (ruled by the twelfth house) for children and babies dying of AIDS. Unfortunately, the place was burned to the ground, probably by local residents who objected to the project. When AIDS was first discovered there was a lot of fear of contagion. Undeterred, Kübler-Ross lectured and gave workshops on AIDS worldwide. Again, the phlegmatic empathy, seeing the larger picture and wishing to stop suffering, would have been her driving force, while her choleric nature would have given her the energy and drive to spearhead her campaign and to not be discouraged by setbacks.

As a phlegmatic, her health was not strong from the outset. Kübler-Ross was born as a triplet and was not expected to live. She did survive, and married, but lost two children to miscarriages, before having two children. In later life Kübler-Ross suffered a series of strokes which left her partially paralyzed. She found living in a wheelchair, slowly waiting for death to come, unbearable. Weakness and collapse are phlegmatic conditions, as is paralysis, and often miscarriages occur because the expulsive faculty is too strong.

Elisabeth Kübler-Ross is a classic phlegmatic, powered by some choler, who responded to suffering with great compassion and brought the reality of death out of the shadows.

Keywords: thoughtful, kind, compassionate, putting others first, physically prone to collapse.

Constitutional remedy: Mouse-Ear (for happiness), Daisy (for wounds from life), Violet (for calm).

Sanguine: Maurice Mességué

Maurice Mességué was a famous French herbalist, who was born in one of the most beautiful regions in France. (Sanguines often live in places of beauty.) His father was a famous local herbalist. Maurice spent an idyllic childhood with him collecting herbs in the beautiful countryside. However, when Maurice was eleven years old his father died (a harsh, melancholic experience). Sent away to school, he was ridiculed and almost friendless; the worst experience for a sanguine is to have no friends. He survived by remembering his long walks with his father and re-creating the countryside in his imagination. Sanguines do bounce back quickly from painful experiences. Their optimism is such that they can find a silver lining in almost any situation, thanks to their natural ebullience, resilience, and imagination. Sanguines are the original positive thinkers, turning lemons into lemonade.

In 1944 Mességué was recruited for the STO or *Le service du travail obligatoire*. The STO was a "deal" between Germany and France: for every three French people who went to Germany to work, one French prisoner of war was released. Mességué was put on the train to Germany; he went into one door of the train and walked out of another. Now a fugitive, he joined the *maquis*, the resistance, and fought for the liberation of France. (Sanguines are quick thinkers, freedom-lovers, and won't be shut in. This cheeky manoeuvre probably saved his life and gave him the opportunity to fight for justice, a cause close to a sanguine's idealistic heart.)

After the war, Mességué became a teacher (a classic sanguine activity). One day he came across a student who was suffering from a severe stomach ache. He gave him plants as a poultice and the student was

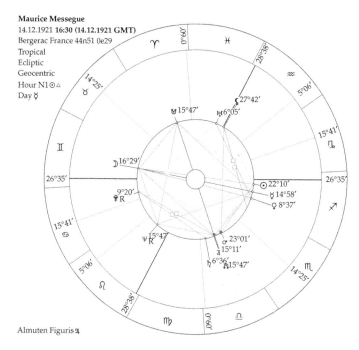

Maurice Messegue
14.12.1921 **16:30 (14.12.1921 GMT)**
Bergerac France 44n51 0e29
Tropical
Ecliptic
Geocentric
Hour N1 ☉ △
Day ☿

Almuten Figuris ♃

Figure 12. Temperament example 3. Maurice Mésséqué. 14 December 1921, 16:38 hrs, Bergerac 44n51 0e29.

	Score	Sanguine	Choleric	Melancholic	Phlegmatic
Temperament of the season	2			2	
Temperament of ascendant sign	2	2			
Temperament of ascendant ruler	1			1	
Temperament of almuten	1	1			
Temperament of Moon sign	2	2			
Moon phase	1		1		
Temperament of Moon ruler	1			1	
	Total	5	1	4	0

cured. Word travelled, and soon Mességué was seeing fifteen patients a week. The headmaster was not amused and told him to stop. Mességué refused, firmly believing he was in the right, especially as he had not charged for his treatments. (Sanguines will always take a stand for what they believe in.) He resigned and settled in Nice to take up his calling as a healer.

> Though my methods were sometimes puerile, I was rediscovering for myself the principle I was to apply for the rest of my life: Treat the patient rather than the disease. (Mességué, 1991, p. 30.)

Mességué had the sanguine's ability to advance far in life due to his genial, friendly nature. He treated the famous actress Mistinguette, who did not pay for her treatment but instead introduced him to her influential friends. Mességué claims to have treated the richest and most glamorous people of the times, including King Farouk of Egypt, poet Jean Cocteau, and Winston Churchill. (Sanguines do like the bright lights of fame and power.) He was also a man of the people and treated a third of his patients for free. (Sanguines are generous and can mix with everyone.)

> Look at lavender, or at nettles or at mint. They are modest-looking plants. One could take them as the very symbols of humility. And yet these three plants alone can deal with as many troubles as can a family medicine-chest full to bursting. (Mességué, 1979, p. 9.)

Mességué was persecuted for practising medicine illegally. (The law and judgement are sanguine activities.) He went to court over twenty times. The publicity these cases generated only enhanced his reputation and gave him the opportunity to demonstrate how skilled a healer he was. (Generating publicity is second nature to Sanguines.) These cases also widened his circle of influence; at his last court case he claimed 20,000 letters had been sent to the Judge in his defence. (Again, showing the sanguine ability to turn the negative into a positive and to attract the support of a wide variety or people.) Mességué warned of the danger of conventional medicine: "I began to realize just how dangerous medicine can be, and when I hear of babies being treated for eczema with shots of cortisone, or year-old infants being given barbiturates, I have no hesitation in calling it criminal folly" (Mességué, 1991, p. 124).

Mességué used his herbs principally in hand and foot baths and poultices (the hands are ruled by Gemini) successfully treating both chronic and acute illnesses. He was very particular about the remedies he used, remembering the fantastic wild meadows of his childhood. Eventually he grew his own organic herbs.

> It was equally clear to me that I couldn't go to some unknown shop in Paris and buy desiccated herbs that would have lost two-thirds of their virtue. I had to have my own plants, I had no confidence in any others. (Mességué, 1991, p. 94.)

Mességué wrote several best-selling books, which were among the first herbals I read. His prose shines out like the warm summer sun and the glorious countryside. He is positive, hopeful, and generous, all sanguine traits. His health is never mentioned, from which we can infer it was as robust as you would expect for a sanguine. His three sixth house planets, Sun, Mercury, and Venus in Sagittarius show tremendous *joie de vivre* and a strong constitution. They also show a man who worked with medicine, in a sunny, generous, open-hearted way.

Keywords: joyful, optimistic, sociable, lucky (or makes own luck), strong physically, resilient.

Constitutional remedy: Melissa (to chill out), Borage (when energy flags).

Melancholic: Dr John Christopher

Like many melancholics, Christopher had a hard start in life. He was born to European parents who left him in an orphanage in Utah. He was later adopted. As a child he suffered from excruciatingly painful rheumatoid arthritis (Saturn rules the bones) and had to walk with a stick or use a wheelchair. He developed hardening of the arteries (Saturn, cold and dry, hardens matter) and croup. Doctors predicted he would die before he was thirty.

Perhaps because of his childhood experiences, after military service he began to treat people with herbs. He studied herbal and naturopathic medicine at several colleges in Canada and the USA (unlike Mességué, who had the sanguine's confidence to use his father's knowledge without formal training).

Dr John Christopher
25.11.1909 5:00 (25.11.1909 12:00 GMT) Salt Lake City, Utah, USA 40°45′39″N 111°53′25″W

Tropical
Ecliptic
Geocentric
Hour N10 ♂ □
Day ♀

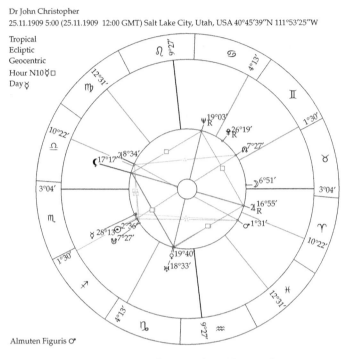

Almuten Figuris ♂

Figure 13. Temperament example 4. John Christopher. 25 November 1909, 05:00 hrs, Salt Lake City 40n46 111w53.

	Score	Sanguine	Choleric	Melancholic	Phlegmatic
Temperament of the season	2			2	
Temperament of ascendant sign	2				2
Temperament of ascendant ruler	1		1		
Temperament of almuten	1		1		
Temperament of Moon sign	2			2	
Moon phase	1		1		
Temperament of Moon ruler	1				1
	Total	0	3	4	3

In 1953 Christopher founded the School of Natural Healing in Utah. Melancholics love to build, organise, and structure. They often need the external validation of public approval, so running a school is an ideal career. Christopher adopted the title "doctor", presumably to give him the gravitas he needed. He became one of the most famous herbalists of his day, creating over fifty herbal formulae which are still available. His school is now run by his son; melancholics like to create dynasties.

Like Mességué, Christopher was repeatedly harassed and prosecuted for practising medicine illegally. But, unlike Mességué, he did not have powerful friends to protect him, or perhaps his melancholy nature did not attract help. Melancholics are often suspicious and distrustful of other people, which makes them more vulnerable to attack. Christopher spent many nights in jail. The Utah Legislature passed a law directed specifically against him, so perhaps his pessimism and suspicion were justified. This law effectively stopped his practice, because the punishment was an indefinite jail sentence (again, the harsh life experience of the melancholic). However, as a determined and ambitious melancholic, Christopher found another way to spread his message. His choleric nature, like that of Kübler-Ross, fought back, and he began teaching and lecturing all over the USA, following a gruelling schedule. (Melancholics love to work hard.) In this way he reached a far wider audience than previously, and attained lasting fame.

Christopher's treatments were what you would expect from a melancholic: severe, drastic, and austere. (Melancholics have an ambivalent relationship with the physical body.) He advocated purges, hydrotherapy, strict naturopathic diets, and heroic doses of medicine. Reputedly, Christopher took three tablespoons of Cayenne in a tumbler of water each morning. His formulas used the locally growing herbs; the formula for adrenal exhaustion contained Mullein leaves, Liquorice root, Cayenne and Ginger root, Hawthorn berries and Ginseng. A deeply religious man (Saturn rules the Abrahamic religions), Christopher died aged seventy-four from an unstated accidental cause. His legacy continues in his school (unlike Mességué, who has a shiny, sanguine website).

Other melancholics: Nicholas Culpeper (see Tobyn, 1997, p. 229).

Keywords: serious, ambitious, inflexible, unlucky (or lacks trust in people and life), physical challenges, pessimist.

Constitutional remedy: Horsetail.

Choleric: Alan Leo

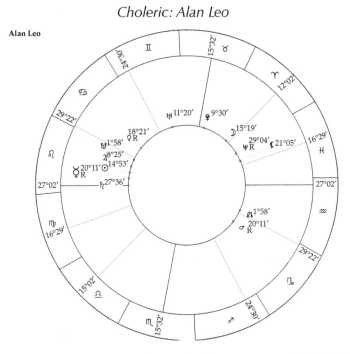

Figure 14. Temperament example 5. Alan Leo. 7 August 1860, 05:49 hrs Westminster 51n30 0w09.

	Score	Sanguine	Choleric	Melancholic	Phlegmatic
Temperament of the season	2		2		
Temperament of ascendant sign	2		2		
Temperament of ascendant ruler	1		1		
Temperament of almuten	1		1		
Temperament of Moon sign	2		2		
Moon phase	1			1	
Temperament of Moon ruler	1		1		
	Total	0	9	1	0

Sometimes called the father of modern astrology, Alan Leo was a classic choleric: dynamic, inspired, and driven. He took the name Leo as a
pseudonym, as it was his Sun sign. He rectified his horoscope to show
his ascendant as Leo rising, a classic choleric move, putting himself centre stage. He was described as:

> a short, thickset man. There was an air of dignity about his personal-
> ity, which tended to make him somewhat proud and self-important,
> but on the other hand he possessed much geniality and there was a
> certain magnetism about his presence … (Curry, 1992, p. 123.)

Leo's geniality masked a formidable will. The choleric neither brooks
nor excuses competition. Choleric does not have the flexibility or mutability of the sanguine, and barges into situations rather than charm his
way in. The choleric is far too impatient to consider other people's feelings, but he is happy for them to bask in his warmth.

Leo wrote that "character was destiny" and moved away from
astrology as divination to it becoming about the personality, the ego,
and identity (all choleric concerns).

> Let us part company with the fatalistic astrologer who prides him-
> self on his predictions and who is ever seeking to convince the
> world that in the predictive side of Astrology alone shall we find its
> value. We need not argue the point as to its reality, but instead make
> a much-needed change in the word and call Astrology the science
> of tendencies. (Curry, 1992, p. 149.)

Pre-destination is anathema to the choleric; they need to believe they
can initiate and create their vision; being passive and powerless against
the fates is unacceptable to them. Leo was a successful businessman.
Interested in the esoteric, after meeting Madam Blavatsky, he became a
Theosophist and learned astrology. He used Theosophy's vast network
to spread his astrological work throughout Europe and America.

Leo started *The Astrologer's Magazine*, later renamed *Modern
Astrology*, using electional astrology[3] to choose the launch date: 20

---

[3]Electional Astrology is the art of choosing the best moment for an event. Traditionally
it was used for battles and coronations (often held at midday so the Sun would be on
the midheaven—its most powerful position. It can also be used for weddings, starting a
business, conferences or significant dates.

July, 1890. Ever the salesman, he offered a free horoscope to subscribers and, in four years, gave away over 4,000 hand-written horoscopes. (Of all the temperaments, choleric has the highest energy.) He also started the Astrology Publishing Company and was hugely successful. Several of his books are still in print, including: *Esoteric Astrology* (1913), *The Key to Your Own Nativity* (1910), and *The Progressed Horoscope* (1906).

In 1915 he founded the Astrological Lodge of London, a branch of the Theosophical Lodge, which continues meeting to this day. All English astrological organizations can trace their roots from the Astrological Lodge: the Astrological Association, the Faculty of Astrological Studies, and the Company of Astrologers. (Cholerics love to initiate, have bold plans, and also the vision and energy to put their ideas into motion.) Leo was no intellectual; he had the cholerics' disdain for theories. He defended himself by saying that one word from the true occultist was worth a thousand of the merely intellectual (Curry, 1992, p. 159).

Leo was dogged by the law. In July 1917 he stood trial for illegally pretending to tell fortunes. He was found guilty and fined £5 and £25 costs, a large sum at the time. Leo declined to appeal but instead set about re-working his whole system to remove any prediction and to focus instead on character analysis (Curry, 1992, p. 157). Compare this to Mességué, who used court cases to promote himself, a true sanguine, and Dr Christopher, who had a punitive experience of the law. Leo took the fine on the chin and set about re-inventing modern astrology. In classic choleric style, Leo threw himself into the work of re-writing, sometimes writing for five hours a day, arguing in true choleric fashion "it must be done quickly, and I must do this myself" (Curry, 1992, p. 158). The strain was too much for him and he suffered a brain haemorrhage and died suddenly in August 1917. It was a typical choleric end: sudden, dramatic and final; there were no lingering goodbyes for him.

Keywords: driven, unsubtle, can-do attitude, leader, egotistical, positive.

Constitutional remedy: Eyebright (to smooth out ruffled feathers), Rosemary (opens the heart), Jack by the Hedge (pure choler; use after setbacks to restore mojo).

Mixed types

Culpeper (1652, p. 58) writes that there are only eight compound temperaments:

1. Choleric-Melancholic.
2. Choleric-Phlegmatic.
3. Melancholic-Choleric.
4. Melancholic-Sanguine.
5. Sanguine-Melancholic.
6. Sanguine-Phlegmatic.
7. Phlegmatic-Sanguine.
8. Phlegmatic-Choleric.

Choleric-Melancholic: Louise Hay

Motivational healer, author, and founder of Hay House Publishing, Hay's book *You Can Heal Your Life* sold over fifty million copies. She had a hard, early life (melancholic) and suffered abuse from her stepfather. She gave birth to a child in her teens, whom she gave up for adoption, and was estranged from her family. In 1970 she was diagnosed with inoperable cancer, which she cured with a regime of forgiveness, therapy, nutrition, and positive psychology (choleric). She founded the Hay Ride for sufferers of AIDS and HIV, and supported thousands of sufferers in the San Francisco Bay area at the height of the epidemic. Hay was already famous and successful but nevertheless took a risk to work with AIDS patients at a time when the disease was feared and marginalised (choleric). She founded the charitable Hay Foundation, which sends her books to prisons in the USA. Hay died peacefully in her sleep, aged ninety. Her choleric nature gave Hay the vision and enthusiasm to embrace the science of mind, and the organisational skills and attention to detail of the melancholic enabled her to run a highly successful publishing company.

Other choleric-melancholics: Starhawk (1-5-4-0).

Culpeper writes of the type:

> They are higher of Stature than such as are Simply Choleric, by reason their radical moisture is more prevalent, yet have they little lean Bodies, rough and hard Skin. Their digestion is meanly strong,

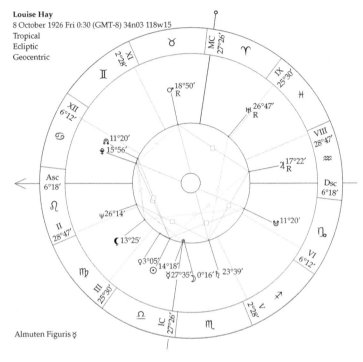

Figure 15. Temperament example 6. Louise Hay. 8 October 1926, 00:30 hrs Los Angeles 118w15.

	Score	Sanguine	Choleric	Melancholic	Phlegmatic
Temperament of the season	2			2	
Temperament of ascendant sign	2		2		
Temperament of ascendant ruler	1		1		
Temperament of almuten	1			1	
Temperament of Moon sign	2				2
Moon phase	1	1			
Temperament of Moon ruler	1		1		
	Total	1	4	3	2

their Pulse meanly strong, yet something slow, their Urine of a pale yellow and thin, their Excrements yellow and hard ... Such people by natural inclination are very quick Witted, excellent Students, yet will they begin many businesses ere they finish one, they are bold, furious, quarrelsome, something fraudulent, prodigal and elo-quent, they are not so unconstant and scornful as Choleric men are, but more suspicious, and fretful, more solitary and studious after Curiosities, and retain their anger longer than Choleric men do. Let them observe great moderation in Meat and Drink, for Meats hard of digestion engenders tough Flegm in such bodies and will bring their Bodies to an Asthma ere they are aware of it. Above all let such people avoid excess in drinking, for much small drink breeds Flegm in them, and much strong spoils the Brain, causeth Scabs and Itch and breaking out of heat about the Body. Moderate Exercise is not only convenient but also very profitable for such persons. (Culpeper, 1652, p. 59.)

Keywords: Leaders, as they both plan meticulously and have vision; quick-thinking, but intolerant of both opposition and slowness; studious, solitary, irritable, more suspicious than choleric and slow to forgive and forget; can be vengeful and bullying (it is interesting that Hay's work focused around forgiveness); ambitious; plays the long game; strong constitution, hard working.

Constitutional remedy: Yarrow for strength and resilience.

Melancholic-Choleric: Leonard Cohen

With the melancholic predominating, life will be harder, the body colder, and digestion weaker. Culpeper writes:

Such are usually tall of stature, yet are their Bodies somewhat slender and dry, their Skin rough, hard, and cold in feeling ... their digestion weak and something less than their Appetite, their Pulse slow, their Urine subcitrine and thin, their egestion sallow colour'd and something thin; dreamings are of falling down from high places, vain idle and fearful things. They are very gentle and sober, willing to do good, admirable students, delighting to be alone, very shamefac'd and bashful, somewhat fretful, con-stant to their Friends, and true in all their actions. Excess of eating, drinking, and sleeping, are as great Enemies to the Nature of such a man ... for they fill the Bodie full of tough and congealed Humors, from whence proceed Morphew and other Infirmities of the Skin, and other Infirmities that are more than Skin deep, as stoppings of the Liver, corruptions of the Lungues, Asthma, Phtisick, Wind, Belly-ach, Chollick ... let them eat and drink moderately, let their care be to suffice Nature and not to stuff their Guts with Meat, nor make a Hog-wash-tub of their Bellies with drink, I will not deny them, but advise them now and then to drink a cup of strong Beer or Wine, especially after meat, for excess of small Beer cools the Liver, hinders their digestion, and bids them beware of a Dropsie, it spoils both Apprehension and Memory, and fills the Head full of superfluities ... moderate Exercise is very good for them, and helps much to destribute vital heat, which in this Complexion seems to be but weak; above all things let them have a care of catching wet at their feet. (Culpeper, 1652, p. 60.)

Keywords: Thoughtful and careful, but less so than a pure melancholic; the choler brings action tempered with planning beforehand; reticence and dislike of the limelight, shy; likes to work behind the scenes, and as an aide rather than a leader; a fine logical mind with intuitive insights; faithful and well-intentioned; prone to depression; likes solitude; strong body, but needs to keep active; poor digestion.

Constitutional remedy: Chamomile (gently warming to the body and emotions).

Leonard Cohen was a Canadian novelist and songwriter-folksinger who became a Buddhist monk. His song "Hallelujah", first released on his studio album *Various Positions* in 1984, became a cult classic recorded by hundreds of artists. Cohen left his fame for a monastic, spiritual life. (Melancholics like to live regulated lives.) Following a period of deep depression (melancholic) in the 70s, Cohen began to embrace Zen. He was introduced by a friend to an elderly Zen teacher. He found the spiritual training rigorous. For a time, he worked in both worlds, the commercial world of music and the spiritual world of striving, until he finally yielded completely and moved to the Mt. Baldy Zen Centre near Los Angeles.

Cohen stopped recording in 1992, touring in 1993, and moved into the Zen Centre in 1994 (melancholic, mountains, solitude, retreat). There he worked on an illustrated book of poems and songs for a future

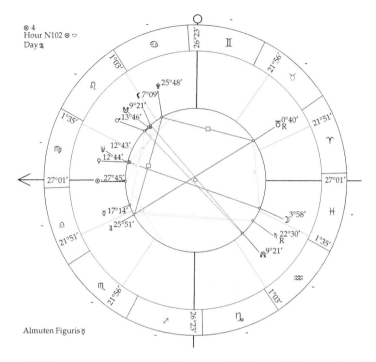

Figure 16. Temperament example 7. Leonard Cohen. 21 September 1934, 06:40 hrs Montreal 73w34 45n31.

	Score	Sanguine	Choleric	Melancholic	Phlegmatic
Temperament of the season	2		2		
Temperament of ascendant sign	2			2	
Temperament of ascendant ruler	1			1	
Temperament of almuten	1			1	
Temperament of Moon sign	2				2
Moon phase	1		1		
Temperament of Moon ruler	1	1			
	Total	1	3	4	2

album. His workroom contained an old computer and a synthesizer, tools for his music and for his graphic art. He rose at 3am for morning meditation and to begin preparing the day's menu. He wrote, "I greet you from the other side of sorrow and despair with a love so vast and shattered, it will reach you everywhere" (melancholic), from the song "Heart with no compassion" on the album *Various Positions* (1984).

Cohen returned to music in 2001. His manager embezzled his money, forcing Cohen to tour again between 2008 and 2010. His choleric nature would have given him the focus and drive to perform and be on stage. He released three albums in the final four years of his life: *Old Ideas* (2012), *Popular Problems* (2014), and *You Want It Darker* (2016), the latter of which was released three weeks before his death. Melancholics embrace old age and many experience a "second flowering" after sixty-five and continue working productively until the end of their lives. Cohen died on 7 November, 2016, at the age of eighty-two, at his home in Los Angeles after a fall. He was suffering from cancer.

Melancholic-Sanguine: Agatha Christie

Culpeper writes of the melancholic-sanguine:

> They are tall of stature, and have big, fleshy, strong bodies, the colour of their Face of a darkish red, their Skin neither hard nor rough, and as little cold, but temperate in respect of softness and warmness … their digestion is good and laudable, their Urine of a light Saffron colour, mean in substance, neither too thick nor too thin, the egestion or Excrements of the Belly reddish and soft, their dreams are pleasant, and many times happen truly to come to pass. They are more liberal, bolder, and merrier than Melancholy persons are, as also less cowardly, not so pensive nor solitary, neither are they troubled with such fearful conceits, but are gentle, sober, patient, trusty, affable, courteous, studious to do others good. For as much as digestion in these is good, they need not be so penurious in Diet as the former, much fasting fill their Bodie full of wind, and much strong Beer and Wine, inflames the Blood. Moderate Exercise purifies their Blood, strengthens their Bodies, and makes their Skin cleer. (Culpeper, 1625, p. 61.)

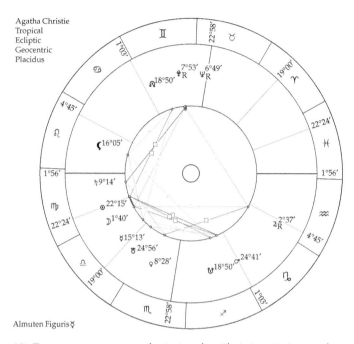

Figure 17. Temperament example 8. Agatha Christie. 15 September 1890, 04:00 hrs Torquay 50n47 3w53.

	Score	Sanguine	Choleric	Melancholic	Phlegmatic
Temperament of the season	2		2		
Temperament of ascendant sign	2			2	
Temperament of ascendant ruler	1			1	
Temperament of almuten	1			1	
Temperament of Moon sign	2	2			
Moon phase	1	1			
Temperament of Moon ruler	1				1
	Total	3	2	4	1

Keywords: Because they are a mixture of opposing qualities, cold and dry and warm and moist, melancholic-sanguines will alternate in how they express their temperament; ability to get on with all types of people and curiosity about life; friendly, but dislike intimacy; analytical minds; love creating imaginary worlds; great game players (non-physical); deep thinkers, but need a social life.

Famous for her novels, Christie had both the melancholic's attention to detail and tight plotting, with the sanguine's light-heartedness and observation of social niceties. She disappeared (melancholic) after her first husband's infidelity was discovered, causing a nationwide hunt for her. Later, she wrote she was suffering from depression and perhaps had a breakdown. Christie later married an archaeologist and spent time working on his digs, cataloguing his finds (melancholic). Her life was a mixture of worldwide fame (sanguine) and retreat. She was a very shy child, and even when famous rarely spoke to the press. But her work has longevity (melancholic). Her play, *The Mousetrap* is the longest running play in the world, opening first in 1952. Her books remain in print and are continuously being filmed. She is said to be the best-selling novelist of all time, having sold around two billion books. She lived quietly in the country until her death in 1976 from natural causes (melancholic).

Keywords: organised and meticulous; ambitious; sociable in the cause of career; thoughtful and intelligent; imagination plus structure.

Constitutional remedy: Melissa (to re-connect with feelings). Agrimony (to find hope and get on with the job).

Sanguine-Melancholic: W.B. Yeats

Culpeper writes:

> They are mean of Stature, but strong well compact Bodies, fleshy but not fat, big Veins and Arteries, smooth warm Skin, something hairy but not so hairy as Sanguine people have: Their Hair is either black or a very black brown, their Cheeks red, something clouded with duskiness, their Pulses great and full, the Urine yellow and mean in respect of thickness and thinness, their digestion good, the Excrements of their Bellies reddish and something thin, they usually dream of deep Pits and Wells and sometimes of flying in the Air. Similar to Sanguine

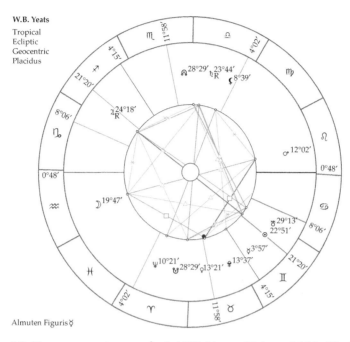

Figure 18. Temperament example 9. W.B. Yeats. 13 June 1865, 22:40 hrs Dublin 53n20 6w15.

	Score	Sanguine	Choleric	Melancholic	Phlegmatic
Temperament of the season	2	2			
Temperament of ascendant sign	2	2			
Temperament of ascendant ruler	1			1	
Temperament of almuten	1			1	
Temperament of Moon sign	2	2			
Moon phase	1			1	
Temperament of Moon ruler	1			1	
	Total	6	0	4	0

but that they are not altogether so merry nor so liberal, a spice of a Melancholy temper being inherent in them. As for Diet and Exercise, that which we described under Melancholly-Sanguine will suffice for these also, only take notice that strong Liquor and violent. Exercise is more subject to inflame the Blood. (Culpeper, 1652, p. 62.)

Keywords: know how to get on with people, but remain distant; similar to sanguine but less sociable and liberal; enjoy pursuits of the mind; disciplined; can create fictional worlds; prefers hierarchies with them at the top.

Constitutional remedy: Rose (to open the heart and deal with disappointments).

Yeats was an Irish poet, dramatist, writer, and occultist, who won the Nobel prize for Literature in 1923. Sanguine-melancholics have both great imagination and the discipline to work at their craft. Yeats was the driving force behind the Irish literary revival and founded the Abbey Theatre (melancholic ambition and sanguine networking). He joined the Golden Dawn and was heavily involved in their magical practices. He was described as courteous and gregarious (sanguine), an intellectual with a strong interest in Irish folklore and history (melancholic). He had a doomed love affair with Maud Gonne, a ravishing Irish revolutionary who introduced him to the Irish Republican cause. Yeats later became a senator in the Irish Free State in 1922. (Melancholics take their responsibilities seriously.) He repeatedly proposed marriage to Maud and was always refused. (Melancholy never giving up with sanguine misplaced optimism.) Yeats has been described as one of the most important poets of the twentieth century. One of his final poems became his epitaph, which I feel encapsulates the sanguine-melancholic dichotomy of optimism versus realism:

> Cast a cold Eye
> On Life, on Death.
> Horseman, pass by.
> (From "Under Ben Bulben" [1938].)

Sanguine-Phlegmatic: Dion Fortune

Culpeper writes:

They are higher of Stature than Sanguine, with strong well set Bodies, not very fat, their Hair is flaxen or very light brown, their

Face is of a paler red, than Sanguine peoples is, neither are their Bodies so hairy, their Pulse is Moderate, their Appetite good, their Digestion indifferent; their Urine subcitrine and mean in substance, their egestion white in some places and red in others, they dream of flying in the Air, Rain and Waters. As for Conditions they are less liberal and not so much addicted to the Sports of Venus as Sanguine are, neither are their Spirits so bold, nor their Bodies so hairy. Seeing the Digestion of such People is but meanly strong, let them not eat as much in one day as they can digest in two, let their Diet be such as is not too hard of digestion, for their Stomachs are nothing never so hot as an Estriches; If they love their appetite better than their health, and will take in more food than is fitting for them, let them expect the Chollick, smal Pox, Meazles, &c. Let not their Drink be too small, for that makes but thin and watry Blood in such Constitutions, it dulls their Brain, and causeth Dropsies and Gouts. Moderate Exercise is very profitable to consume their Superfluities. (Culpeper, 1652, p. 63.)

Keywords: Mutable and changeable, they can fit into any situation; inconstant, they change their views often and seek out novelty; lassitude and indolence, seeing easy solutions; easy-going and friendly, kind hearted and sensitive; less bold and liberal than sanguine.

Constitutional remedy: Vervain (for tenacity).

The Temperament is equally mixed sanguine and phlegmatic (4:0:2:4).

Because they are both moist temperaments, sanguine-phlegmatics are elusive and inconstant. They shift positions and can easily adapt to different situations. They can be multi-talented (like Leonardo da Vinci) and move from project to project effortlessly. They have good people skills (sanguine) but need solitude (phlegmatic). Fortune was a novelist, high magician, and the foremost female figure in twentieth century occultism. Known to those in her inner circle as "DF", her pseudonym was inspired by her family motto *Deo, non-fortuna* (Latin for "by God, not fate"), originally the ancient motto of the Barons and Earls Digby. She was responsible for the cult of Glastonbury in the inter-war years. She founded the Society of the Inner Light, (phlegmatic spiritual seeking) which continues to operate and was heavily influenced by Alice Bailey's ideas. After her death a breakaway group formed Dolores Ashcroft-Nowiki's Servants of the Light in Jersey. Vivienne Crowley claimed Fortune was a proto-Wiccan and

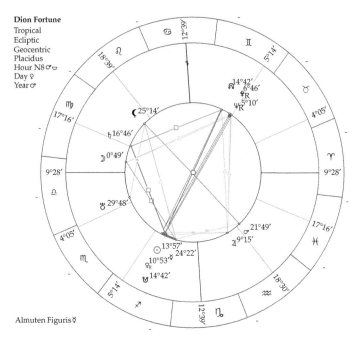

Figure 19. Temperament example 10. Dion Fortune. 6 December 1890, 02:11 hrs Llandudno 53n19 3w49.

	Score	Sanguine	Choleric	Melancholic	Phlegmatic
Temperament of the season	2			2	
Temperament of ascendant sign	2	2			
Temperament of ascendant ruler	1				1
Temperament of almuten	1				1
Temperament of Moon sign	2	2			
Moon phase	1				1
Temperament of Moon ruler	1				1
	Total	4	0	2	4

was pivotal in the development of the feminist Wiccan movement in the 1970s and 1980s, whose luminaries include Starhawk, author of *The Spiral Dance* (1979), and Marion Zimmer Bradley, author of *The Mists of Avalon* (1983) and founder of the Aquarian Order of the Restoration. Dion Fortune died of leukaemia in 1946, aged fifty-five (a disease of the blood—sanguine).

Phlegmatic-Sanguine: Leonardo da Vinci

Culpeper writes:

> Phlegmatic-Sanguine people are but mean of stature, somewhat gross and fat of Body, smooth soft Skin, and somewhat cold in touching, they have but few hairs upon their Bodies and are long without Beards, their hair is light yellow, light brown or flaxen, no waies curling, their colour whitely, with some very small redness, if any; their digestion is somewhat weak and less than their Appetites, their Pulse small and low, their Urine somewhat thick and pale-ish, they sometimes dream of falling down from some high place into the water. Their Conditions are so-so, between Phlegmatic and Sanguine, neither very liberal nor very covetous, neither very idle nor much employed, neither very merry nor very sad; rather fearful of the two than valiant. Let them beware of overfilling themselves with meat, if they love their health but half so well as they love their ease so they will; much eating and drinking fills the Stomachs of such people full of raw humors, and sour phlegm, engenders the small Pox and Measles, and dulls their wit, which naturally is none of the quickest. Strong Beer and Wine taken in Mediocrity is not hurtful for them, and let them take this from me, and say I told them the truth, the more they accustom their Bodies to exercise, the better 'tis for them. (Culpeper, 1652, p. 64.)

Keywords: social butterfly; imaginative and creative; open-minded and changeable; relaxed and untroubled; lazy and unmotivated; fearful rather than brave.Constitutional remedy: Shepherd's Purse (for boundaries).

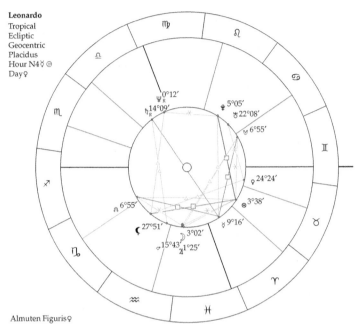

Figure 20. Temperament example 11. Leonardo da Vinci. 14 April 1452, 21:40 hrs Vinci, Italy 43n47 10e55.

	Score	Sanguine	Choleric	Melancholic	Phlegmatic
Temperament of the season	2	2			
Temperament of the ascendant sign	2		2		
Temperament of the ascendant ruler	1	1			
Temperament of almuten	1				1
Temperament of Moon sign	2				2
Moon phase	1				1
Temperament of Moon ruler	1				1
	Total	3	2	0	5

Phegmatic/Sanguine 5:3.

Leonardo shows the soaring mind of the phlegmatic-sanguine. He was responsible for some of the most sublime art of the Renaissance: the Mona Lisa, the Last Supper, the Adoration of the Magi (phlegmatic aesthetic and spiritual sensitivity). However, many of his paintings were unfinished (phlegmatic slowness, laziness, and dislike of endings). He was interested in mechanics, predicted and designed an airplane, a submarine, a machine gun and a tank (sanguine curiosity and love of puzzles). He courted and was patronised by the powerful, including the Borgias, the Medicis, the Duke of Milan and Kings Louis XII and Francis I of France (sanguine love of power and ease of finding powerful friends). His homosexual lifestyle brought him into conflict with the law in Florence. Luckily, one of his co-defendants was the son of a wealthy nobleman and so the charges were dismissed (sanguine luck, phlegmatic slipperiness). The public disapprobation, however, spurred Leonardo to travel abroad and find other wealthy patrons (sanguine turning of negative experiences into positives). He worked with mathematician Luca Pacioli, proving the divine proportion and, while under the patronage of Pope Leo X, conducted many scientific experiments.

He had an unusual lifestyle, was a vegetarian, and reputedly would buy caged birds so that he could set them free (sanguine need for freedom) (Vasari, 1965, p. 257). In his will (Vasari, 1965, p. 258–9) he left money to pay for sixty beggars to follow his casket to its final resting place (phlegmatic concern for the underdog). Leonardo is recognised as the archetypal Renaissance man. He was a musician, engineer, painter, sculptor, cartographer, mathematician, philosopher, botanist, and anatomist, which typifies sanguine curiosity, the airy need need to systematise and understand how things work.

Phlegmatic-Choleric: Ram Dass

Culpeper writes:

> Such are tall of stature but not so big nor yet so fat as phlegmatic, their Bodies are something hairy and they pretty soon have Beards, they have usually Hair of a Chestnut colour, not curling, and soft, their Faces of a tawny red, full of Freckles, their

Appetite and Digestion is indifferent, as being pretty well met; a moderate and pretty full Pulse, their Urine subcitrine and mean in respect of thickness, the Excrements of their Belly of a pale yellow and thick, they usually dream of swimming in the Water, Snow, and Rain. They are not such drowsy, lazy, sleepy Creatures as phlegmatic folks are, but are nimbler, bolder, and kinder, merrier, and quicker witted. Although they may be a little bolder with their food than phlegmatic may, yet is digestion in them none of the strongest, and excess in meat fills their Bodies with Choler, and punisheth their Carcasses with Choleric Diseases. Excess of Drink spoils their Digestion, and weakens Nature, but moderate Exercise refresheth it. (Culpeper, 1652, p. 65.)

Keywords: less slow than phlegmatics, quicker, bolder, merrier and quick-witted; kinder than choleric; inspired and sensitive; driven and reclusive; energetic and lazy; daring and shy; slow to anger but fierce when roused.

Constitutional remedy: Lavender (to calm down) and Speedwell (for inspiration).

Ram Dass is an American-born spiritual teacher, former academic, and clinical psychiatrist (melancholic) and author of the classic spiritual text *Be Here Now* (1971) (melancholic and down-to-earth). Originally named Richard Alpert, he was an associate of Timothy Leary at Harvard in the 1960s where they used hallucinogens in psychological experiments with students. They were both fired from Harvard and founded a psychedelic community in Mexico (choleric). Alpert split with Leary, found a spiritual teacher, and took the name Ram Dass. He founded the Seva Foundation to treat the blind in developing countries and work on reforestation projects and health education for the Dakota tribe (phlegmatic). He became a personal carer to his father and urged service on his followers. He worked with the homeless and set up a hospice for the dying (phlegmatic). He raised over $500,000 in a sixty-city lecture tour for his charities (choleric). Following a stroke he became paralysed, which, he wrote, gave him the gift of silence (phlegmatic).

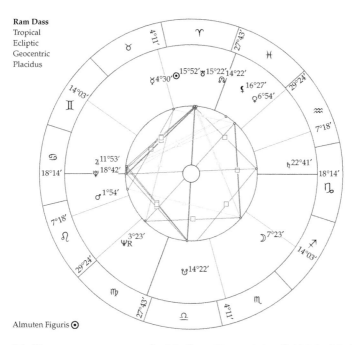

Figure 21. Temperament example 12. Ram Dass. 6 April 1931, 10:40 hrs Boston 42n22 71w04.

	Score	Sanguine	Choleric	Melancholic	Phlegmatic
Temperament of the season	2	2			
Temperament ascendant sign	2				2
Temperament of ascendant ruler	1				1
Temperament of almuten	1		1		
Temperament of Moon sign	2		2		
Moon phase	1			1	
Temperament of Moon ruler	1	1			
	Total	3	3	1	3

Choleric-Phlegmatic: Jonathan Cainer

Culpeper writes:

> Such are but mean of stature, but stout lusty strong Bodies, strong
> Bones, well set Creatures, neither fat nor lean, but in that respect
> they keep the Golden Mean, they have lusty great Bones, their Skin
> is hairy and moderate to feeling in respect of heat and moisture,
> their Hair is yellowish or sandy flaxen, and their Face of a tawny-
> ish yellow colour, their Digestion is good, their Pulse swift, their
> Urine thin and of the colour of Saffron, their egestion yellow and
> hard, they dream of fighting, Lightning and Rain, hot Baths and
> hot Waters. Their Conditions are not much different from those of
> Choleric men, only the Vices of Choler is moderated by Phlegm,
> therefore a Choleric-Phlegmatic man is nothing so vicious as one
> purely Choleric; neither doth any Humour set a stop to the unbri-
> dled passions of Choler, so as Phlegm doth, because 'tis so contrary
> to it, judge the like by the rest. A slender Diet works the same evil
> effects in quality though not in quantity that it doth in Choleric.
> Much excess in strong Drink inflames the Blood, and out of such
> Inflammation proceeds Putrefaction, which begets a Generation of
> rotten Fevers. (Culpeper, 1652, p. 66.)

Keywords: Similar to choleric but more moderate and less aggressive;
likes attention but needs solitude; active and impulsive sometimes,
inactive other times; will feel out the answer to problems; extreme and
then conservative; selfish and humanitarian. High energy followed by
collapse. Spiritual and pragmatic.

Constitutional remedy: Daisy (for when they bump into life). Borage
and Oat straw (for burnout and emotional healing).

Johnathan Cainer, astrologer, was the highest-paid journalist on
the *Daily Mail*, a newspaper whose politics he despised. (Choleric-
phlegmatics are both unconventional and pragmatic.) He fell into astrology by accident, when someone drew up his natal chart, and he was
impressed by its accuracy. (Phlegmatic trusting his instincts.) He studied at the Faculty of Astrological Studies and was the first to develop
a computer programme for astrologers. (Cholerics are always ahead of
the game.) He was a philanthropist who supported the Steiner School

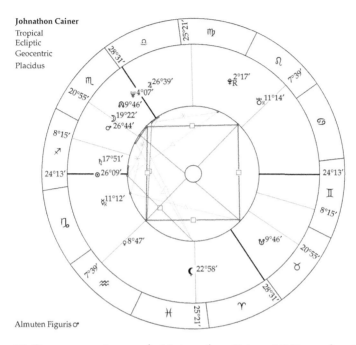

Figure 22. Temperament example 13. Jonathan Cainer. 18 December 1957, 08:00 hrs London 51n30 0w10.

	Score	Sanguine	Choleric	Melancholic	Phlegmatic
Temperament of the season	2			2	
Temperament of ascendant sign	2		2		
Temperament of ascendant ruler	1	1			
Temperament of almuten	1		1		
Temperament of Moon sign	2				2
Moon phase	1				1
Temperament of planet ruling Moon sign	1		1		
	Total	1	4	2	3

in New York (phlegmatic). He moved between newspapers to get the coverage he wanted (choleric looking out for number one), and was the best-known astrologer in the UK. His first wife died suddenly in an accident (choleric) and he was left to care for his six children (phlegmatic). He died suddenly of a suspected heart attack aged fifty-eight, possibly drug-related (choleric).

Of course, small, potted biographies cannot give the whole picture of a person's life, but I hope these examples will show how the different temperaments are expressed. The self-confidence of the choleric, the optimism of the sanguine, the compassion of the phlegmatic, and the hardworking melancholic are, I believe, easily recognizable everywhere. All these virtues are needed in the world: vision without compassion becomes tyranny; structure without energy ossifies; feeling without action changes nothing; and action without forethought is dangerous. The temperaments may explain why blanket dietary advice is not suitable for everyone: the phlegmatic needs less cold food, while the choleric needs more; similarly, exercise for a sanguine should be moderate, while for a melancholic it is vital to keep the energy moving. Temperament may also explain why certain remedies may not work on certain people, despite their traditional use for the condition in question, while constitutional remedies will give support to the healthy body.

As I said when discussing the elements, the temperaments are seen through our eyes as westerners and carry the baggage of a culture that values the mind (sanguine) above the feelings (phlegmatic) and is institutionally misogynist and racist. Herbalist Richard Whelan (2011) has an interesting take on the temperaments: he has assigned them to animals, thereby discarding their dubious origin in slave-owning Ancient Greece and incorporating them into a worldview which embraces everyone. Feel free to do the same; the essence of the temperaments may be better described in another guise. But that is another story.

AFTERWORD

This book started with Greece in the sixth century BCE and has travelled to the twenty-first century. Today there is a small revival of interest in these traditional techniques among Western herbal practitioners who are looking for a holistic philosophy within which to practise their art. Like medicine post-Enlightenment, herbal medicine is dogged by *scientism*, by which I mean applying scientific methods to areas that cannot be reduced to objective measuring. Clinical trials on various herbs do add to the body of knowledge and give herbalists a boost when encountering scepticism and ridicule from various interest groups. But herbal medicine cannot be reduced to mechanistic science any more than mainstream medicine can, and have still have a positive outcome.

Dr Lown in his book *The Lost Art of Healing* (1999). Makes a plea for the art of healing to be restored to its central place in the art of medicine. Medical students, he maintains, should be schooled in the humanities before biomedical sciences to develop sensitivity and compassion. He writes of the importance of touch, rather than checking vital signs, and working with the patient as a whole person, not as a collection of systems, and using words to bolster the patient's vitality and capacity to deal with the lifestyle stressors that are contributing to the sickness.

Herbalists, because they are increasingly trained in university science departments, can fall prey to this mechanistic, piecemeal approach, by using herbs good for x or y, rather than taking in the totality of the patient as a complex, multi-faceted individual. The discipline of traditional diagnosis helps to see the larger picture where the practitioner and patient engage in a dialogue about how best to address their problems and heal the whole person, body, emotions, and spirit.

What, then, for the future? We are lucky in the UK that we do not send our herbalists to jail, nor our astrologers, but herbalism remains a poor relation in the shiny world of complementary medicine. However, in recent years herbal medicine has been at the heart of another movement, which Culpeper would have approved of: radical herbalism. Below, I outline several grassroots movements to bring herbal medicine to the dispossessed.

Herbalists Without Borders, Bristol

This is a collaboration between clinical herbalists, community herbalists, herb growers, and local migrant support projects. They are a branch of Herbalists Without Borders UK, which is affiliated with the International Herbalists Without Borders.

Setting up a clinic is a deeply rooted act of resistance against an unjust global political system that has created such unjust borders, as well as the government's introduction of the Immigration Act 2016, which exacerbates the already extreme difficulties refugees and asylum seekers are facing.

Homelessness, unstable housing, poverty, loneliness, and social isolation, whilst living in a constant state of uncertainty regarding their future and asylum status, are just some of the challenges that people who have fled their homes face daily. Living in such stressful conditions greatly impacts their health.

Herbalists Without Borders believe that herbal medicine is an important part of any healthcare system and can have profound effects individually, as a community, and in wider society. Current projects include: a mobile dispensary for common ailments such as insomnia, anxiety, coughs, and low immunity; the dispensary is taken to existing support projects in the city. They run a free herbal clinic where people needing more in-depth support can access one-to-one consultations with trained herbalists. Lastly, they are involved in the harvesting of herbs from local growing projects with migrants.[1]

Calais and Dunkirk

Herbalists Without Borders have also been working at the refugee camps in Calais and Dunkirk, to provide medicine and first aid remedies to these very vulnerable people. After the camp in Dunkirk was burned down, funds were raised for a mobile women's centre.

Herbal Unity, Glasgow

The Herbal Unity Collective[2] was set up in Glasgow in late 2015, in response to changes in legislation that restricted access to healthcare among people without immigration papers. The collective is comprised of clinical and lay herbalists, people in the asylum process, massage therapists, growers, and grassroots campaigners. Their politics are aligned with The Unity Centre and No Borders.

They believe that healthcare is a right and not a privilege and should be freely accessible to all people. They aim to achieve this by providing alternatives in the form of a grassroots, free-to-access, patient-centred herbal clinic. They believe that herbal medicine is not only effective, but removes our reliance on the pharmaceutical industry, which is a hierarchical, capitalist system that degrades our environment and our autonomy over our own health.

More than just access, they stand for a healthcare system that recognises diversity, where people can have choice and control over what forms of medicine or other healing practice they wish to use.

They view health holistically, seeing it as made up of our physical, mental, and psycho-emotional selves, but also, they look beyond the individual to the root causes of ill-health in the social, political, and environmental injustices of our society.

They have an anti-oppressive approach to healthcare provision and actively challenge the patient-doctor paradigm, instead working collectively to empower us to feel we have more control over our own health.

---

[1]Herbalists Without Borders, Bristol website: https://bristolhwb.org.
[2]Contact email address: unityherbalclinic@gmail.com (September, 2018).

They actively challenge racism, sexism, classism, ableism, homophobia, transphobia, capitalism, patriarchy, and institutions that exploit, neglect, and degrade us. Police and representatives of the Home Office are not welcome in their clinic space.

Since the collective formed, the project has grown rapidly due to demand. The clinic offers: a drop-in herbal dispensary, herbal consultations and follow-ups, massage, hot food, childcare, herbalism, and a self-care library. They also run a monthly herbal study group, open to all, and a gardening group to develop a medicine garden outside of the space. With so many people using the clinics the cost of repeat herbal medicine has been an ongoing concern. To help with some of the costs they have been growing and foraging as much of the medicine used as possible. They have been making, oils, tinctures, balms, and creams for the clinic. These activities, as well as providing some of the stock for the clinic, have created an atmosphere of self-care and empowerment for people to access their own medication. They have organised a training weekend to share skills and make volunteering at the clinic accessible to anyone who is interested.

Not much has changed. As Culpeper commented in 1651:

> I wish from my heart our present State would take this matter into consideration and take a little care for the lives of the poor Commonalty, that a poor man that wants money to buy his wife and Children bread, may not perish for want of an angel to fee a proud insulting domineering Physitian, to give him a Visit. I think it is a duty belonging to the Keepers of the Liberty of England I would help my poor brethren in this particular if I could, but I cannot. (Culpeper, 1651a, p. 172.)

Grass Roots Remedies Co-operative

Another Scottish project offering holistic care within a NHS framework, the Grass Roots Remedies Co-operative runs The Herbal Clinic, a low-cost integrated herbal clinic within the NHS Wester Hailes Healthy Living Centre, staffed by two fully qualified Medical Herbalists, offering herbal consultations to local residents for a donation of whatever they can afford, not turning anyone away for lack of funds. Herbal medicines are prescribed for free.

Treating a wide range of health complaints, the demographic of the client base means they support patients presenting with: anxiety, low mood, clinical depression, addiction and withdrawal, recovery from trauma and abuse, digestive issues, hormonal issues, chronic pain, auto-immune disease, cancer, and bereavement. With excellent results so far, the reputation of the clinic is spreading. They treat refugees and asylum seekers who can't access mainstream medical services and take referrals from local doctors. Since 2015, they have seen 200 patients and had 600 repeat visits, despite only being open one day a week. They have also now received referrals from three other doctors' practices, and have received encouraging letters from consultants in local neurology and renal departments.

Their ethos is person-centred, accepting people's life circumstances without judgement, working with care to respect and support autonomous choices, and contributing to long-term social change by providing vital services to the marginalised. They also refer patients to free counselling, food co-ops, free cookery classes, support groups, massage, gym memberships and access to a grow-your-own community garden. A herb growing project called CommuniTea is supporting community gardens, schools, and individuals to grow crops of different herbs, to harvest and process them as blended herbal teas for free distribution around the neighbourhood. They have been heartened to find nurses, doctors, and health visitors amongst their supporters.[3]

In the UK, healthcare operates within the framework of the NHS, which, for all its failings, provides a safety net for most people. However, perhaps State medicine is a mixed blessing. I know from my experience of treating patients over the last forty years that the mixture, complexity, and sheer number of drugs that patients are prescribed has increased exponentially, with little benefit to overall health and wellbeing, and sometimes with alarming side effects.

Although no friend to alternative medicine, Ben Goldacre (2012) wrote a book exposing the conflict of interest within the pharmaceutical industry that has corrupted medicine. Goldacre describes how pharmaceutical companies selectively release the results of medical trials, those revealing side effects tending to be withheld.[4] Recently in the news is

---

[3]Grass Roots Remedies website: www.grassrootsremedies.co.uk.
[4]Dr. Richard Horton, writing in *The Lancet*, commented: "The case against science is straightforward: much of the scientific literature, perhaps half, may simply be untrue. Afflicted by studies with small sample sizes, tiny effects, invalid exploratory analyses, and flagrant conflicts of interest, together with an obsession for pursuing fashionable trends of dubious importance, science has taken a turn towards darkness" (Horton, 2018, p. 1380).

the spiraling use of opioids in England (Boseley, 2018). The prescription of opioids is steadily rising even though they are highly addictive and ineffective for chronic pain. And more sinister is that a study in the *British Journal of General Practice* found that ninety per cent of these prescriptions were in deprived areas in the North of England. The opioid epidemic in the USA is well-documented and is the reason life expectancy has fallen there for the first time in a century (Erickson, 2017).

The Republic of Ireland does not have a National Health Service. Herbalist Vivienne Campbell spoke to me in a personal communication about what that means for health and wellbeing in the Republic. Fees are quite high and prescription costs can run to a hundred euros or more for a course of antibiotics. I was quite shocked at this, being a child of the NHS myself, but I wondered what the effect on the health of the people was, and how this affected their choice of treatment. Unsurprisingly, Campbell suggested that people took better care of themselves and that, if you have to pay, you paid more attention to what you spent your money on. This was especially true of infections, such as cystitis or chest infections, which often recur despite repeated rounds of antibiotics. For this reason, herbalists in the Republic of Ireland enjoy a popularity lacking in the UK, where herbalists compete with free NHS treatment. Also, in Ireland there is the tradition of "cures" where each family has its own expertise in healing a particular condition, and so the folk memory of using herbs for health is strong.

Clearly, a free NHS is wonderful for accident and emergency treatment, and for certain acute illnesses, but it may be argued that the healing arts advocated by Dr Lown are trampled underfoot by Big Pharma and its greed for profit. Campbell sees a future in Ireland for a herbal hospital, which could sit easily beside orthodox medicine. Indeed, in the past hospital doctors used herbal remedies successfully (Quinlan, 1883). Switzerland has an integrated healthcare system, with thirty per cent of people with chronic health conditions having consulted an alternative practitioner (Klein et al., 2015), which may provide a template for the future.

To finish, here is a speech from the opening plenary at the Radical Herbs Gathering, 2016:

> The word Radical comes from the *radix* Latin word for "root". As Herbalists we often promote ourselves as getting to the root cause of illness and taking a wholistic perspective that differs from the reductionist view of allopathic medicine.

At this gathering we ask if we are really getting to the root cause of ill health and taking a wholistic perspective if we treat someone, physically, emotionally and spiritually but we do not consider the environmental, social and political factors which cause disease?

For health is intrinsically linked to our eco systems and society. Capitalism directly or indirectly harms and oppresses people, makes them ill while the environment is poisoned for profit. Can we really say we are getting to the root cause or taking a wholistic perspective if we don't challenge or resist these structures and institutions?

When I was at university there was lots of talk about how to charge £50 an hour, setting up business and valuing our time, and while it is true we must make a living, there was never any discussion that herbal medicine is private medicine. How do we make herbal medicine accessible and serve our community as a herbalist while offering medicine to people who can't afford to pay us? There was never any talk of how to organise and survive as herbalists/health practitioners in a world where our free medicine is dominated by a multi-billion pound pharmaceutical industry.

True healing is about responsibility. Responsibility means responding by whatever means available to care for our communities and our environment and to respond to the current global humanitarian crisis with the diverse skills we have. If politics affects everyone in their life, then the personal is political and healing is political. Planting a tree is revolutionary, seed bombing and guerrilla gardening are revolutionary, organic gardening is revolutionary.

We must be aware of our privilege in the western world; just because we don't see direct oppression and harm, it doesn't mean it doesn't exist. It's important we identify with the struggle, find the struggle, and walk alongside the people who really suffer; remembering our privilege in the western world is at the expense of others. As we build a new paradigm, remember the words of Grace Lee Boggs, "I don't know what the next revolution will look like, but you could imagine it, if your imagination was rich enough".

Let's challenge and resist the systems that oppress us while we re-build our communities from the bottom up. Let's focus on the action part of non-violent direct action and reclaim the heart of humanity for each one of us. (Naylor, 2016, personal email communication.)

Or, as Culpeper wrote four hundred years ago:

> I am well aware, that he, who stands forward to promote the
> public welfare at the expense of a particular profession, must excite
> enmity, and draw upon him the clamour of interested individuals.
> But the solid comfort resulting from a sense of doing good, and
> the reflection of becoming instrumental in preserving the health of
> thousands, surpasses the fleeting praises of the multitude, or the
> smiles of self-exalted and ambitious men. (Culpeper, 1798, p. xvi.)

I would like to finish with these chilling words, written by Plato in the
fourth century BCE:

> There are two kinds of medicine. Medicine for slaves and medicine
> for people. Medicine for slaves must remove symptoms fast, so they
> can go back to work. Medicine for the people tries to understand
> the symptom and its meaning for the body as a whole, in order to
> restore balance and harmony. (Bury, 1967–8, line 720c).[5]

---

[5]The exact text reads: "the slave doctor neither gives nor receives any account of the several ailments of the domestic [slave] but prescribes what he deems right from experience." While the freeborn doctor treats freemen "by investigating them ... according to the course of nature." Suggesting the quick-fix medicine for the poor/slaves and holistic medicine for those who can pay for it.

APPENDIX 1

Working magically with plants

This is how I began working this way with plants and how I still run my groups today. If you are alone, you may wish to record this journey first and then play it to yourself. For the best experience, use freshly picked plants. Dried will work but are less strong.

Find a space where you will not be disturbed for thirty minutes or more. Sit or lie and feel comfortable and warm enough.

First take the plant and hold it in your hand. Look at it, really look at it closely. Look at the structure of the plant, how it is put together. Look at the leaves and flowers or root. What do their shape and colour tell you about the plant? Is it strong or delicate, brightly coloured or pale? Its size and strength may tell you something about its personality, how it grows, where it grows, what kind of environment it flourishes in. Then taste the plant, allow the flavour to fill your taste buds. As you taste it, be aware of any sensations in your body, any memories or images the taste evokes. Be aware of the flavours of the plant. Some have an initial flavour followed by a different one. Again, notice the effect the flavours have on your mouth.

Then, going a little deeper, close your eyes and turn your eye inwards and downwards and focus in on the emotional nature of the plant. If this plant were a person, what kind of person would they be? What would their character be? How would they dress? How would they walk into a room? What would their energies be like? Check out any feelings that come up; where in your body do you feel them? Allow any images or memories to come up and remember them, and then let them go without judgement. Going deeper in, feel the heart of this plant, their essence. Allow them to envelop you, enfold you, and absorb you. Follow where the images lead you. They may make no sense to you, but just allow them. Remember them and then let them go.

Get a sense of how this plant would be used ritually. Would it be used in a group context or would you use it alone? Get a sense of what type of ritual it would be appropriate for.

Then, going deeper still, allow the plant spirit to approach you. It may be a person, an animal, or an image or feeling, but allow them to approach and greet them. Register their appearance, and especially look closely into their eyes. Allow the spirit to dialogue with you. It may use words or images, or you will get the sense or meaning of what they are trying to communicate. Allow them to lead you deeper into the essence of the plant and follow and register what they show you.

Spend five or ten minutes with the spirit and then, slowly reverse back, going through the ritual uses, notice any new information that comes up. Then the emotional uses, and then the physical uses. Before you leave, gain a clear sense of the temperature of this plant, the planet it is governed by, which chakra it is associated with, how best to take it—tea, tincture, bath, etc.—and what time of day, and what season. Finally, what kind of person it would suit the best, and who you would not give it to, and why.

Slowly come back into the room and write down what you found out.

Herbs, planets and temperaments

	Herbs of the Sun	*Herbs of the Moon*	*Herbs of Mercury*	*Herbs of Venus*	*Herbs of Mars*	*Herbs of Jupiter*	*Herbs of Saturn*
Hot 1st	Eyebright St. John's Wort Chamomile	Cleavers	Liquorice Coriander Fenugreek Valerian	Ox Eye Mallow Marshmallow Rose Cowslip	Basil	Borage Burdock Agrimony Avens Almond Bugloss Chervil	Coriander
Hot 2nd	Saffron Rosemary Cinnamon		Lavender Fennel Dill White Horehound Parsley Senna	Vervain Motherwort Ground Ivy Archangel Mugwort	Wormwood Hops Holy Thistle	Lemon Balm Milk Thistle Betony Sage	
Hot 3rd	Juniper Rue Angelica Celandine Centaury		Lavender Honeysuckle Elecampane White horehound	Mint Thyme Pennyroyal Feverfew White dead nettle	Nettle Ginger Vitex	Meadowsweet	

(*Continued*)

	Herbs of the Sun	Herbs of the Moon	Herbs of Mercury	Herbs of Venus	Herbs of Mars	Herbs of Jupiter	Herbs of Saturn
Hot 4th			Jack by the Hedge		Garlic Onion Leeks		
Cold 1st				Violet Rose Yarrow Plantain Coltsfoot Oats			Comfrey Shepherd's Purse
Cold 2nd		Lettuce Chickweed Willow				Dandelion	Fumitory
Cold 3rd							Bistort Nightshade
Cold 4th		Poppy Hemlock					Henbane Mandrake
Moist 1st	Marigold	Cleavers Mouse ear Speedwell	Liquorice Valerian	Mallow Coltsfoot Archangel	Basil	Borage Bugloss	

Moist 2nd		Lettuce chickweed purslane poppy cucumber	Fennel	Violet Marshmallow Daisy		Meadowseet Wood betony	
Moist 4th		Chickweed					
Dry 1st	Chamomile Saffron Juniper St John's Wort Eyebright Agrimony	Cleavers	Fenugreek	Cowslip Coltsfoot Rose		Burdock	Shepherd's Purse
Dry 2nd	Rosemary		Fennel Valerian Lavender	Ladies Mantle Vervain	Hops Wormwood	Betony Dandelion Sage	
Dry 3rd	Celandine Angelica		Honeysuckle Elecampane Lavender		Ginger	Meadowsweet	
Dry 4th					Garlic Onion		

Five emollient herbs

Marshmallow, Mallow, Violet, Beets, Pellitory.

Four cordial flowers

Borage, Bugloss, Rose, Violet.

Four greater hot seeds

Anis, Caraway, Cumin, Fennel.

Four lesser cold seeds

Succory, Endive, Lettuce, Plantain.

Purges choler

Groundsel, Hops, Peach Leaves, Wormwood, Century, Mallow, Senna, Barberry, Hops, Violets, Damask Rose. Barley water, raisins, prunes.

Modify the belly in choler: Sorrel, Lettuce, Mallow, Spinach, cherries, apples, peaches.

Purges phlegm

Hyssop (Oxymel), Elder flowers, Bryony, Broom. Coriander water, Fenugreek with honey. Loosen the belly in phlegmatic cause: Oatmeal, beets, Marigold leaves.

Purges melancholy

Fumitory with honey and water, Ox Eye Daisy, Senna.

Purges heart: Lemon Balm, Rosemary, Bugloss, Borage.

Stomach: Wormwood, Mint, Fennel, Chervil, Thyme, Marigold, Radish, vinegar.

Liver: Wormwood, Century, Agrimony, Fennel, Endive, Hops.

Spleen: Wormwood, Watercress, Thyme.

Kidney and bladder: Nettles, Rocket, Elecampane, Burnett, Saxifrage, Pellitory of the Wall.

Lungs: Lemon Balm, Holy Thistle.

Symptoms

A hot and dry brain

A cause of continual Headaches, and the more it exceeds the golden Mean in heat and driness, the greater is the pain. Remedies of such a distemper of the Brain, use, Fumitory, Willow Leaves, Lettice, Hops, Water Lillies, white Poppy Seeds, Roses, Violet Leaves and Flowers, Strawberry Leaves, the Seeds of Endive, Succory, Musk-Millions, and Pumpions, you may use them which way you please they are all harmless. (Culpeper, 1652, p. 22.)

A hot and moist brain

There follows a high colour of the Face, the Eyes are hot and burning, and look red, the Veins of the Temples seem great, the excrements of the Head are many, yet seem well concocted, all hot things whether taken inwardly or applied outwardly cause them to have a stretching distention and heaviness in their Head, if you moisten their Heads they avoid excrement the more Roots of Parsley, the Roots and Leaves of Fennel, Mugwort, Plantane, Vervain, and Willow Leaves are good Medicines, they may boyl them in Water and drink the Decoction. (Culpeper, 1652, p. 22.)

A cold dry brain

If a distemper of cold and driness afflict the Brain, the Face is cold in feeling, livid, swarthy and discoloured to the Eye, you can see no Veins in their Eyes, and their Head is easily afflicted both by cold, and cold things; the temper of their Brain and Head is very unequal, for some times their Heads are light and excrements flow thence moderately, sometimes they are exceedingly troubled with heaviness of their Heads. Such whose Brains are cold and dry, have admirable Memories, and are fantastick in their actions, fearful, and think everything they do, whether it be Meat or Drink, or Exercise of Body, doth them harm, they sleep very badly &c. Such people are very subject to Lethargies, Coma, Carus, and other Diseases of the Head that proceed of coldness and moisture.

For Cure, Juniper Berries are excellent to eat ten or twelve of them every morning fasting; as also Bettony, Chamomel, Peony

Roots and Seeds, Calaminth, Fennel, sweet Marjoram, Pennyroyal, Mother of Time &c. (Culpeper, 1652, p. 24.)

Signs of a hot and dry heart

If the Heart be oppressed with heat and driness, the Pulses are great, hard, and swift, they fetch their Breath swiftly, and the swifter if the breadth of the Breast answer not equally by proportion to the heat of the Heart, their Breast is very rugged if they be sick, but if it be natural to them, it is very hairy, they are full of action, hasty in all things, angry and Tyrannical. Herbs Medicinal for such as labour under this Infirmity, are, Borage, Bugloss, Sorrel, Wood-sorrel, Lettice, Purslane, &c. these and Syrups or Conserves made of them. (Culpeper, 1652, p. 33.)

Signs of a hot and moist heart

If moisture together with heat predominate at the Heart, the Man's Breast is not so tough nor hairy, they are quick enough to anger and Action, but not so cruel in their anger as if driness prevail, their Pulse is great, soft, swift, and frequent: If the Breast be large they draw their Breath very deep, if narrow, very thick, and their experation or letting out their Breath, is done with more swiftness than their inspiration or drawing in their Breath, such Bodies are mighty subject to Diseases of Putrefaction of Humors. Things Medicinal for such, are Conserves of red Roses, Syrup of Violets, of Bawm and of Citron Pils, as also of the Juyce of Citrons and Lemmon. As for Simples, Citron Seeds, Rue, Bawm, Angelica Roots and Leaves, Wood-sorrel, the Flowers or Roses, Borrage, Bugloss, and Violets; (above all sweating may be commended in this infirmity). (Culpeper, 1652, p. 34.)

Signs of a cold and moist heart

Indications of the Heart when coldness with moisture abounds, are softness of the Pulse, Fearfulness of Mind, slowness of Body, he hath scarce Spirit enough to be angry, much less to fight; as for such things as belongs to the Breast and the rest of the Body you may distinguish them as you were taught before. Much exercise is very convenient for such Bodies, I suppose there were but few troubled with this infirmity in the Spartan Common-wealth in Lycurgus his time, Thrashing, and cleaving Logs is good Physick for them [that is, vigorous exercise. I recommend dancing for the exercise-averse]. For Simples, Rue, Angelica Roots, Nutmeg, Cinnamon, Saffron, Marigold Flowers, Betony, Balm, Elecampane, Rosemary Leaves and Flowers. (Culpeper, 1652, p. 35.)

Signs of a cold and dry heart

The Heart being cold and dry renders the Pulse hard and small, yet respiration, if the smallness of the Breast answer to the coldness of the Heart, is moderate, if the Breast be very Broad 'tis bare and slow, above all men these are least prone to anger, but once anger them and they will never care for you more, there is not one of a hundred of them that hath any Hair of his Breast. Conserves of Roses, Borage, Bugloss, and Rosemary Flowers is very good for such; as also Marigold Flowers, Saffron, green Walnuts preserved, Juniper Berries, Betony, Candied Citron Pills. (Culpeper, 1652, p. 36.)

Signs of a hot and dry liver

The Indications of the Liver when it is hotter and drier than it ought to be, are, The Bowels are rough, the Blood thick and dry, soundly pestered with Choler, it is yellow Choler in youth, but black or addust Choler in age, the party is subject to dry Scabs, the Veins are large and hard, and although the Heat of the Heart may withstand the coldness of the Liver, yet cannot the moisture of the Heart withstand the dryness of the Liver, for the dryness of the Heart is sooner overcome by the moisture of the Liver, than the dryness of the Liver by the moisture of the Heart. Herbs Medicinable are Liverwort, Strawberry and Violet Leaves, Raisons of the Sun, Endive, Succory, Fumitory, Water-Lillies, Lettice, Purslaine, Nightshade, these or any of these, or others like them in operation, are excellent to boil in clarified Whey in the Summer time. Also, the Compounds of them, Syrups or Conserves made of them: as also Dandelion, Scabious, Devils bit, Scurvy-grass, Groundsel, Peach Leaves, Dyers Weed, Furs Flowers &c. (Culpeper, 1652, p. 41.)

How many wayes our Bodies may be altered

1. Air [pollution].
2. Motion and rest, both of the whole Body, and of every part thereof.

3. Sleeping and watching [insomnia].
4. Meat and Drink.
5. Excrements of the Body.
6. Affections of the Soul. (Culpeper, 1652, p. 87.)

Culpeper on emotions

Affections of the Mind, and they are but two, Content, and Discontent.
    In Content, consider,

1. What it is.
2. Its Effects.
3. Its Differences.

First, By Content, I mean such affections as are pleasing to the Nature of Man, as Hope, Joy, Love, Mirth, & c.
    Secondly, By their Effects;

1. They dilate the Heart and Arteries.
2. They distribute both Vital and Natural Spirit throughout the Body.
3. They comfort and strengthen not only the parts of the Body, but also the Mind, and that in all their actions.

Thirdly, Their Differences are two and no more.

1. Moderation, which comforts both Body and Mind.
2. mmoderation, which hurts both Body and Mind.

First, By Discontent, I mean such affections as disturb the Body, as Anger, Hatred, Fear for things to come, Care for things past, Sorrow, Grief of Mind & c.
    Secondly, The Effects of it are,

1. They divert the Vital heat from the Circumference to the Center, thereby consuming the Vital Spirits, drying the Body and causing Leanness.
2. They are forerunners of Evil.
3. They are Destroyers, Overthrowers and Murderers both of Body and Mind.
4. They hasten old Age and death by consuming Radical Moisture. (Culpeper, 1652, p. 100.)

APPENDIX 2

Chart of elements and temperaments

Element	Physical	Emotional	Mental	Spiritual
Fire	Athletic	Irritable, driven	Inspired, unsubtle	Ecstasy
Earth	Bony, wiry	Pessimistic, introvert	Scientific, logical	Earth Magic
Air	Youthful	Optimistic, extravert	Quick, superficial	Meditation
Water	Fleshy soft	Fearful, sensitive	Rambling, psychic	Bliss, union
TEMPERAMENT				
Choleric	Muscular, strong	Restless, angry	Intuitive, rash	Spiritual warrior
Melancholic	Stooping	Resentful, careful	Focused, thoughtful	Service

(*Continued*)

Element	Physical	Emotional	Mental	Spiritual
Sanguine	Larger than life	Joyful, self-assured	Optimistic Boastful	Pranayama
Phlegmatic	Slow	Compassionate	Dreamy	Sacrifice
PLANETS				
Sun ☉	Regal	Warm, joyful	Clear thinking	Raja Yoga
Moon ☽	Retiring	Gentle, kind	Compassionate	Psychic
Mercury ☿	Youthful	Cool, logical	Superficial	Mind
Venus ♀	Voluptuous	Passionate	Collegiate	Love
Mars ♂	Hot	Impatient, bombastic	Incisive	Courage
Jupiter ♃	Large, warm	Positive	Philosophical	Higher mind
Saturn ♄	Sparse, cold	Suspicious, responsible	Deep thought	Orthodox religions

Simplified table of Ptolemy's planetary dignities

This is a quick guide to see where planets are happy (well-placed) and where they are weak. In the astrology section we discussed which planets ruled which signs, but the planets are also exalted (very strong) or in detriment (weak) and in fall (weakest) in certain signs. The signs also have rulers in the day and night, which are sometimes the same (Cancer, Scorpio, Pisces) or different planets (Virgo, Capricorn, etc.)

This is a simplified table. The entire table also contains the terms and faces, which are the degrees in each sign that the planets rule. To my mind this is an added layer of complication, but others do use them.[1]

---

[1]For the full table of Ptolemy see Lilly, 1647, p.104.

Sign	Ruler	Exalted	Day	Night	Detriment	Fall
Aries ♈	Mars ♂	Sun ☉	Sun ☉	Jupiter ♃	Venus ♀	Saturn ♄
Taurus ♉	Venus ♀	Moon ☽	Venus ♀	Moon ☽	Mars ♂	–
Gemini ♊	Mercury ☿	–	Saturn ♄	Jupiter ♃	Jupiter ♃	–
Cancer ♋	Moon ☽	Jupiter ♃	Mars ♂	Mars ♂	Saturn ♄	Mars ♂
Leo ♌	Sun ☉	–	Sun ☉	Jupiter ♃	Saturn ♄	–
Virgo ♍	Mercury ☿	Mercury ☿	Venus ♀	Moon ☽	Jupiter ♃	Venus ♀
Libra ♎	Venus ♀	Saturn ♄	Saturn ♄	Mercury ☿	Mars ♂	Sun ☉
Scorpio ♏	Mars ♂	–	Mars ♂	Mars ♂	Venus ♀	Moon ☽
Sagittarius ♐	Jupiter ♃	–	Sun ☉	Jupiter ♃	Mercury ☿	–
Capricorn ♑	Saturn ♄	Mars ♂	Venus ♀	Moon ☽	Moon ☽	Jupiter ♃
Aquarius ♒	Saturn ♄	–	Saturn ♄	Mercury ☿	Sun ☉	–
Pisces ♓	Jupiter ♃	Venus ♀	Mars ♂	Mars ♂	Mercury ☿	Mercury ☿

REFERENCES

Because Culpeper's books have been in print since their publication, there are many, many versions, particularly of *The English Physician*, some of which exclude the astrology. Other authors have added their own thoughts into the text, which may or may not be helpful. The best versions to consult are online at the Wellcome Institute and university libraries, such as: https://quod.lib.umich.edu and https://archive.org.

Appleby, D. (1985). *Horary Astrology*. Wellingborough: Aquarian.

Arroyo, S. (1978). *Astrology, Psychology and the Four Elements*. Davis, CA: CRCS.

Barton, T. (1994). *Ancient Astrology*. London: Routledge.

Brooke, E. (1993). *Women Healers Through History*. London: Women's Press.

Brooke, E. (2018). *A Woman's Book of Herbs*. London: Aeon.

Bury, R. G. (trans) (1967–8). *Plato in Twelve Volumes. Vol. X & XI.* Cambridge Mass: Harvard University Press.

Chadwick, J., & Mann, W. N. (1950). *The Medical Works of Hippocrates*. London: Blackwell.

Cornelius, G. (1994). *The Moment of Astrology: Origins in Divination*. London: Arkana.

Culpeper, N. (1649). *A Physical Directory or Translation of the London Dispensary*. London: Peter Cole.

Culpeper, N. (1651a). *Semeiotica Uranica*. London: John Booker.

Culpeper, N. (1651b). *Ephemeris for 1651*. London: Peter Cole.

Culpeper, N. (1652). *Galen's Art of Physick*. London: Peter Cole.

Culpeper, N. (1653). *Pharmacopoeia Londinensis*. London: Peter Cole.

Culpeper, N. (1789). *Culpeper's English Physician and Complete Herbal*, edited by E. Sibly. London: British Directory Office.

Culpeper, N. (1806). *The English Physician Enlarged*. Manchester: S. Russell.

Curry, P. (1992). *A Confusion of Prophets: Victorian and Edwardian Astrology*. London: Collins & Brown.

Emoto, M. (2004). *The Hidden Messages in Water*, trans. D. Thayne. New York: Atria.

Gawrońska-Grzywacz, M., et al. (2011). Biological activity of new flavonoid from Hieracium pilosella L. *Open Life Sciences*, 6(3): 397–404.

Gerard, J. (1636). *The Herball or Generall Historie of Plantes*. London: Adam Islip. Book 2, chapter 312, page 852

Goldacre, B. (2012). *Bad Pharma: How Drug Companies Mislead Doctors and Harm Patients*. London: Forth Estate.

Goodrick-Clarke, N. (1999). *Paracelsus: Essential Readings*. Berkeley, CA: North Atlantic.

Greenbaum, D. G. (2005). *Temperament: Astrology's Forgotten Key*. Bournemouth: Wessex Astrologer.

Grieve, M. (1977). *A Modern Herbal*. London: Penguin.

Gullan-Whur, M. (1987). *The Four Elements*. London: Rider.

Gunther, R. T. (1968). *The Greek Herbal of Dioscorides*. New York: Hafner.

Hippocrates (1868). *Airs, Waters and Places*. Edited and translated by W.H.S. Jones. Cambridge, MA: Harvard University.

Hippocrates (1975a). *Aphorisms*. Edited and translated by W.H.S. Jones. Cambridge, MA: Harvard University.

Hippocrates (1975b). *Regimen for Health*. Edited and translated by W.H.S. Jones. Cambridge, MA: Harvard University.

Hippocrates (1979a). *Laws*. Edited and translated by W.H.S. Jones. Cambridge, MA: Harvard University.

Hippocrates (1979b). *The Nature of Man*. Edited and translated by W.H.S. Jones. Cambridge, MA: Harvard University.

Horton, R. (2018). Offline: what is medicine's 5 sigma? *The Lancet*, 385: 1380.

Houlding, D. (2007). Virgo the maiden. *The Mountain Astrologer*, 134: 25–31.

Iyengar, B. K. S. (1974). *Light on Yoga*. London: Mandala.

Leo, A. (1911). *The Astrologer and his Work*. London: L.N. Fowler.

Liddell, H. G., & Scott, R. (1944). *Liddell and Scott's Greek-English Lexicon*, abridged version. Oxford: Clarendon.

Lilly, W. (1647). *Christian Astrology* [reprinted London: Regulus, 1985].

Lilly, W. (1715). *The Last of the Astrologers: Mr William Lilly's History of His Life and Times from the Year 1602 to 1681*. Second edition, edited by K.M. Briggs [Reprinted London: Folklore Society, 1974].

Lown, B. (1999). *The Lost Art of Healing: Practicing Compassion in Healing*. New York: Ballantine.

Mességué, M. (1979). *Health Secrets of Plants and Herbs*. London: Collins.

Mességué, M. (1991). *Of People and Plants*. Rochester, VT: First Healing Arts.

Nutton, V. (2013). *Ancient Medicine*. Abingdon: Routledge.

O'Donohue, J. (2010). *The Four Elements*. London: Transworld.

Ogilvie, B. W. (2006). *The Science of Describing: Natural History in Renaissance Europe*. Chicago: University of Chicago.

Parker, D., & Parker, J. (1983). *A History of Astrology*. London: Andre Deutsch.

Quinlan, F. J. B. (1883). Galium aparine as a remedy for chronic ulcers. *British Medical Journal, 1172*: 1173–1174.

Radice, B. (1973). *Who's Who in the Ancient World*. London: Penguin.

Riddle, J. M. (1985). *Dioscorides on Pharmacy and Medicine*. Austin, TX: University of Texas.

Robbins, F. E. (Ed.) (1940). *Tetrabiblos*. Cambridge, MA: Harvard University.

Said, E. W. (1978). *Orientalism: Western Conceptions of the Orient*. New York: Pantheon.

Sarton, G. (1959). *A History of Science*. Cambridge: Cambridge University.

Tester, J. (1987). *A History of Western Astrology*. Woodbridge: Boydell.

Tobyn, G. (1997). *Culpeper's Medicine: a Practice of Western Holistic Medicine*. Shaftsbury: Element Books.

Toomer, G. J. (1985). Galen on the astronomers and astrologers. *Archive for History of Exact Sciences, 32*(3/4): 193–206.

Vasari, G. (1965). *Lives of the Artists*. Translated by G. Bull. London: Penguin.

Watson, L. (1971). *Supernature*. London: Hodder and Stoughton.

Woodward, M. (Ed.) (1636). *Gerard's Herball: The Essence Thereof Distilled*. London: Thomas Johnson [reprinted London: Minerva, 1971].

Zoller, R. (1989). *The Arabic Parts in Astrology: the Lost Key to Prediction*. Rochester, VT: Inner Traditions.

Websites

Boseley, S. (2018). Prescription of opioid drugs continues to rise in England. *Guardian*, 13 February. Available at: www.theguardian.com/society/2018/feb/13/prescription-of-opioid-drugs-continues-to-rise-in-england.

Devlin, H. (2018). Mixing herbal remedies and conventional drugs "could be harmful". *Guardian*, 24 January. Available at: www.the-guardian.com/science/2018/jan/24/mixing-herbal-remedies-and-conventional-drugs-could-be-harmful.

Erickson, A. (2017). Opioid abuse in the US is so bad it's lowering life expectancy. *Washington Post*, 28 December. Available at: www.washingtonpost.com/news/worldviews/wp/2017/12/28/opioid-abuse-in-america-is-so-bad-its-lowering-our-life-expectancy-why-hasnt-the-epidemic-hit-other-countries.

Gilliam, F. (2007). The ecological significance of the herbaceous layer in temperate forest ecosystems. *BioScience, 57*: 845–858. Available at: academic.oup.com/bioscience/article/57/10/845/232416.

Grass Roots Remedies (2018). grassrootsremedies.co.uk. Accessed: September, 2018.

Herbalists Without Borders, Bristol (2018). https://bristolhwb.org. Accessed: September, 2018.

Joseph, R. (2018). Doctors, revolt! *New York Times*, 24 February. Available at: www.nytimes.com/2018/02/24/opinion/sunday/doctors-revolt-bernard-lown.html.

Klein, S. D., Torchetti, L., Frei-Erb, M., & Wolf, U. (2015). Usage of complementary medicine in Switzerland: results of the Swiss health survey 2012 and development since 2007. *PLoS ONE, 10* (10). Available at: https://doi.org/10.1371/journal.pone.0141985.

Macfarlane, R. (2016). The secrets of the wood wide web. *New Yorker*, 7 August. Available at: www.newyorker.com/tech/elements/the-secrets-of-the-wood-wide-web.

Maciocia, G. (2015). Lecture on gui: ghosts and spirits in chinese medicine. https://youtu.be/fBlYNSDNX3I. Accessed: September, 2018.

RobGMacfarlane. (2018). Word of the day: "Chelidonias". https://twitter.com/robgmacfarlane/status/988296534663024640. Accessed: September, 2018.

Tree Sisters (2010). treesisters.org. Accessed: August, 2018.

Wellcome Collection (2018). Botanical encounters. wellcomecollection.org/events/botanical-encounters. Accessed: August 2018.

Whelan, R. (2011). Introduction to constitutional medicine. http://www.rjwhelan.co.nz/articles/constitutional_medicine_introduction.html. Accessed: September, 2018.

INDEX